MEDICINAL
PLANTS
OF NIGERIA
An Ethnobotanical Survey and Plant Album

MEDICINAL
PLANTS
OF NIGERIA
An Ethnobotanical Survey and Plant Album

ANSELM ADODO, OSB

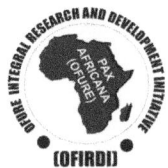

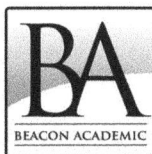

PAX AFRICANA (OFURE)
OFURE INTEGRAL RESEARCH AND DEVELOPMENT INITIATIVE
(OFIRDI)

BA
BEACON ACADEMIC

First Published in 2018
By OFIRDI and Beacon Academic

Ofure (Pax) Integral research and Development initiative (OFIRDI)
Plot 74A, Sir Michael Otedola Crescent off Joel Ogunnaike street, by
Lagos Country Club, GRA, Ikeja. Lagos. info@paxafricana. +234 706
744 0203 www.paxafricana.org

Beacon Academic, Innospace, Chester Street, Manchester, M1 5GD, UK
www.beaconbooks.net

ISBN: 978-1-912356-16-4

Cover design by Bipin Mistry
Image by Rawpixel and Chua Bing Quan on Unsplash

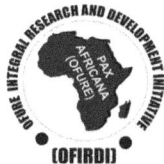

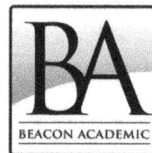

Table of Contents

Acknowledgements

The successful completion of this book is a result of collective efforts by a team of dedicated researchers at Paxherbal clinic and research laboratories (Paxherbals). Emmanuel Amodu, curator at Paxherbal herbarium and Austin Obi, our photographer, travelled to different parts of the country, even to remote and dangerous places, to identify and take photographs of plants that were once common but have become scarce. Tunde Owolabi and Kingsley Ezenwa, research scientists at Paxherbals, were involved in the time-consuming qualitative aspect of this research work. There are over eighty staff members of Paxherbals who contributed in one way or another to this research work. Space and time will not allow me to mention their names individually. My sincere appreciation goes to them all.

Foreword

The book by Reverend Father Anselm Adodo, titled Medicinal Plants of Nigeria – An Ethnobotanical Survey and Plant Album is a "must read" for those desiring to learn more about the role of plants in the prevention and treatment of major disease conditions. Being an orthodox medical practitioner and a researcher myself, I have observed the tendency for persons affected by the disease to ask questions about alternative treatment remedies based on the use of plant products. The frequent answer has always been that there is limited information about the basis for the use of plants and their derivatives for the treatment and prevention of various diseases, while some medical practitioners actually discourage their patients from using plant-derived products. Nevertheless, it is common knowledge that despite these suggestions often made by orthodox practitioners, the use of plants for the treatment and prevention of ailments in various parts of the world, especially in sub-Saharan Africa has continued unabated. By contrast, several governments including the Nigerian government and the World Health Organization have identified the untapped potential in plants for resolving some of the most pressing health challenges facing humankind, and have recommended further research and systematic documentation into medicinal plant products.

Indeed, there is abundant evidence that many of the solutions to diseases are locked away in plants. Some medications currently used in orthodox medical practice are derivatives of plants. Over 100 active ingredients are presently known to be derived from plants for use as drugs and medicines. These include medications such as aspirin derived from willow bark, penicillin from Penicillium mold, cocaine from the coca plant, and quinine used for the treatment of malaria that is derived from a tree native to South America. As reported by Dr. Anselm Adodo in this book, of the 400,000 species plants in the world, about 25% (100,000 species) are used in various continents for the treatment and prevention of diseases. Among the 100,000 species of potentially medicinally beneficial plants, only 10,000 (10%) have been clinically analyzed and categorized for human consumption. Additionally, the fact that many of the recommendations made for the prevention of diseases such as cancers, hypertension and cardiovascular diseases emphasize the use of plant-based products including natural fruits, vegetables, and foods with high fiber content, suggest that there are active biologically active ingredients that are available in these plants that may not have been thoroughly investigated.

Thus, ignorance about the origin, nature, and nomenclature of medicinally useful plants largely accounts for the misinformation and the current poor understanding of the role that plants can play in the treatment and prevention of diseases. This book contributes to resolving this challenge by documenting the plants that are used traditionally for the treatment of local disease conditions in Nigeria and elucidating their origins, history, taxonomy, and ethno-pharmacognosy. Although the book is mainly focused on Nigerian products, it has implications for other parts of sub-Saharan Africa and the developing world where information about similar products are also highly limited. The book sits apart from others in using a community-based approach which enables readers to relate to the traditional practice of herbal medicine as the bedrock of the practice of ethnomedicine in our part of the world. Without such an approach, there would be a missing link which would not allow documentation of the full extent of the use of plants as medicinal products. The generational gulch which has not permitted the uptake of ethnomedical practice by the younger generations of the originators of medicinal plant products further justifies the use of the community-based approach in developing the book.

Father Dr. Anselm Adodo has many years of experience in research and use of traditional plants as medicinal products. He is one of the leading progenitors and a "Master in the Act" of medicinal plants in our part of the world. His work at the Pax Herbal Clinic and Research Laboratories (popularly called Paxherbals) in Ewu, Esan Central Local Government Area of Edo State, Nigeria, has come with immense national and international reputation. The Paxherbals is, without doubt, the most accepted and widely acclaimed Centre for medicinal plants in sub-Saharan Africa, which is visited annually by thousands of pilgrims seeking solutions to various ailments. As a witness to the public defense of his Ph.D. by the Da Vinci Institute, South Africa, I can testify to Dr. Adodo's scientific creativity and inventiveness, his keen sense of community discovery and resourcefulness, and his leadership and high knowledge in the field of ethnomedicine.

In sum, I am convinced that this book makes a substantial contribution to providing new knowledge about medicinal plants native to the southern part of Nigeria. It is written with high fluidity, academic sophistication and profound intellectual acumen. I am extremely delighted that Father Dr. Adodo has been able to find time from his busy pastoral duties to document his experiences in great detail in the new book. I recommend the book very highly to students, academics, community leaders, policymakers and all those who believe in examining the untapped potentials of medicinal plants for the improvement of health in various parts of the world.

Prof. Friday E. Okonofua,
BSc (Hons.) (Ile-Ife), MB ChB (Ile-Ife) Ph.D. (Karolinska), FRCOG ed audem, FICS, FMCOG, FWACS, FAS
Professor of Obstetrics and Gynaecology,
And Vice-Chancellor, University of Medical Sciences,
Ondo City, Ondo State, Nigeria

Preface

It has taken seventeen years for this book to become a reality. Since the publication of *Nature Power* in the year 2000, there has always been a demand for a subsequent book of this kind, so as to help readers identify the medicinal plants pictorially. When *Nature Power* was first published, at the time, the practice of herbal medicine in Nigeria and in most parts of Africa was mainly, and widely associated with witchcraft, sorcery, ritualism and all sorts of nativefetish practices and beliefs. Because of the fact that herbal medicine was highly linked to paganism, therefore, many African Christians decided to secretly patronize traditional healers, while the elites and the religious figures did not want to identify in any way with traditional African Medicine, not at any one point even. The *Nature Power,* therefore, like a lonely voice in the wilderness, was written to try and correct the misconception that African Herbal medicine is synonymous with paganism, ritualism, and fetishism. Seventeen years after its publication, the levels of negative perceptions have reduced considerably. Since then, people from all walks of life, namely; religious authorities, medical practitioners, healthcare professionals, academics, etc now openly and proudly patronize herbal medicine and speak boldly in support of it. There is also a growing interest at the moment in the scientific study of herbal medicine across the continent, and Nigeria in particular.

University of Medical Sciences (UNIMED), Ondo, the only university of its kind in Nigeria is in the process of introducing a bachelor's degree program in Herbal Medicine into its curriculum. This is historic, and a very important step towards boosting herbal medicine research and development in Nigeria. It is in recognition of this that I asked the Pioneer Vice-chancellor of UNIMED, Prof. Friday Okonofua, professor of Gynaecology and Obstetrics, to write the foreword to this book.

Samuel Adegboyega University, Ogwa, a private University in Edo State is also in the process of introducing a degree programme in Herbal Medicine into its curricula through the inspiration of its Vice Chancellor, Prof. Bernard Aigbokhan. The University of Ibadan has already approved and commenced a Master's degree and a Ph.D. in African Traditional Medicine at its Institute of African Studies, while a course in herbal medicine, through the Pharmacy department, has already been introduced into the medical curriculum at the same university. An expert committee, with members drawn from government research and regulatory agencies, set up by the Standards Organization of Nigeria (SON) to draw up standards for official identification of African medicinal plants, has also made huge progress in its research findings by this time.

The Nigeria Institute of Medical Research (NIMR), recently also established a Centre for Herbal Medicine, Alternative and Complementary Medicine Research. The Nigeria Natural Medicine Development Agency (NNMDA), together with the Pax Herbal Clinic and Research Laboratories (PAXHERBALS) have already prepared a detailed protocol for a clinical trial of the Pax herbal malarial medicine called Malatreat, which is awaiting ethical clearance from health regulatory authorities. At the same time, the Federal Institute of Industrial Research, Oshodi (FIIRO), Nigeria has signed a memorandum of understanding with PAXHERBALS to carry out research into the use of Nigerian plants as foods and medicine, with a view of commercializing the products.

These are some of the exciting developments in the area of herbal medicine research in Nigeria. And in all these instances, I have always been actively involved, either as a member of a curriculum advisory committee, curriculum review committee or a research committee. My participation brought awareness to several areas of neglect, especially the dearth of literature on herbal medicine from Nigeria and documentation of Nigerian plants and flora for students and researchers. This has compelled Nigerian researchers to depend excessively on foreign publications to help them in their local research, which is practically difficult and not easy to compare. It is therefore important for African scholars to publish their research findings to save the situation, otherwise, we will perpetually continue to depend on research data from abroad, mainly: Asia, Europe, and America.

It is also important to note that traditional healers have become a highly endangered species, as many of them die mainly due to old age and other tropical diseases, without passing on their knowledge and expertise to their children and grandchildren. This has all been facilitated by the high rate of migration of the immediate generation to the cities, in the quest for modern education, where they attend modern universities and acquire degrees in fields like modern medicine, business administration, banking, architecture, geography, criminology, engineering, and a host of others. Some become fire-spitting evangelists, pastors and Christian crusaders who declare 'war' on traditional medicine and brand their own kinsmen, as idol worshippers and pagans. Western education and foreign religions seem to have indoctrinated African children against their predecessors, traditions, and culture, which has led to the current dimness in knowledge, as far as traditional medicine is concerned. I sincerely hope that the curricula in Herbal Medicine contribute greatly towards solving this quagmire.

One of the major weaknesses of Traditional Medicine, however, is that it has not yet moved from the realm of the subjective to the objective as well as implicit to explicit knowledge. It is thus crucial, that traditional medicine evolves from implicit to explicit knowledge, from knowledge embodied in individual local healers to a community of knowledge that is available to all.

In Africa, it is often difficult to separate the practice of herbal medicine as a discipline, from the personality of the herbal practitioner. In conventional medicine, it is different; if a patient dies after a series of treatment and medication, people rarely blame or condemn the practice of medicine as a discipline, or declare it completely ineffective. Rather, it just means that a particular case was simply impossible, or not successful. If a Medical doctor makes mistakes or acts contrary to the principle of "doing no harm", or is noticed to have been negligent, he or she is penalized by the relevant authorities. However, such individual mistakes and inefficiencies do not always mean that the discipline of medicine is bad, and the people understand. On the contrary, people often fail to make this distinction when it comes to traditional medicine, they often judge and condemn the practice of herbal medicine itself when an individual practitioner defaults or is negligent. This is partly due to lack of a strong control and regulatory system as well, that ensures discipline and effectiveness. On the other hand, lack of documentation, illiteracy and little emphasis on knowledge sharing and research, has greatly retarded traditional medicine as a field of discipline.

My greatest wish is that this book encourages other African scholars to publish their work. It is important that we preserve the vast body of our indigenous knowledge in writing, thereby making it explicit so that it can be passed on to others.

Introduction

This book aims to serve as a workbook for students, teachers and practitioners in the field of ethnobotany and ethnomedicine. It documents the plants that are traditionally used by the local population, the history of local use, and the traditional beliefs around the use in Nigeria. At a time when so much attention is being given to phytochemical screening of plants, there is a temptation to overlook the philosophy of ethnomedicine and cultural use of plants, thereby losing the link between plants and the community. This research adopts a community-oriented approach to African herbal medicine research and argues for a return to a community-based approach to medicine, wherein the health of the individual is closely aligned with that of the community. Community in this context includes plants, animals and the environment.

There are two approaches to the practice of herbal medicine: a clinic-oriented approach and a community-oriented approach. In the clinic oriented approach, emphasis is placed on scientific identification, conservation and use of medicinal plants. Laboratory research and screening are carried out to determine plants' chemical composition and biological activities. Great interest is shown in quality control of raw materials and finished products, and in the development of methods for large-scale production of herbal drugs, which are labelled and packaged in the same way as modern drugs. They are also distributed through similar channels as modern drugs, that is, through recognised health officials in hospitals, health centres or pharmaceutical supply chains. The government, private companies and non-governmental organisations invest relatively huge sums of money in promoting further research in herbal medicine. In the clinic-oriented approach, minimal interest is shown in the socio-cultural use of the plants (LeGrand and Wondergem, 1990).

In the community-oriented approach, the emphasis is on the crude and local production of herbs to apply simple but effective herbal remedies to common illnesses in the local community. Knowledge of the medicinal uses of herbs is spread among community members to promote self-reliance, and information is freely given on disease prevention and the origin of diseases. No interest is shown in mass production of drugs for transportation to other parts of the country or exportation to other countries. The cultural context of the plants used is taken into account, and local perceptions of health and

1

healing often takes precedence over modern diagnostic technology. Simple herbal recipes are used for the treatment of illnesses such as coughs, colds, catarrh, malaria, typhoid and ulcers.

The approaches outlined above are two extremes of the same reality. There is a need to harmonise these two extremes to complement each other, as there seems to be little cooperation between the people working on either side. Scientists, pharmacists and medical doctors who follow the clinic-oriented, exogenous approach tend to sneer at and look down on traditional health practitioners. Meanwhile, traditional healers closely guard their indigenous knowledge and refuse to reveal their formulae and production systems to the so-called professionals. This inevitably leads to herbal medicine practitioners being labelled as "secretive", "esoteric" or "unscientific" (Adodo, 2017).

There is a third approach, which this book endorses: a return to the indigenous way of thinking, though in modern guise, that transcends the dichotomies between man and woman, nature and humans, community and the individual. This is a return to a transdisciplinary, transcultural, transpersonal and transformational mode of knowledge creation – an evolution so to speak – from the traditional academic confines of University to the more open "Communiversity", a community of knowledge that emerges from and is fully grounded in nature and community. The uniqueness of this research lies in its open-minded approach to science as a product of the community in which it grows, and as something that should serve the needs of that community. This matters, because if research is disconnected from the community it leads to a "dis-eased" research outcome – such as a botanist and a taxonomist who, while gaining a technical knowledge of trees and plants, have lost knowledge of the forest, or the astronaut who, while becoming an expert in the study of the moon and the stars, has lost knowledge of the sky.

A study of the history of medicine in Europe shows that medicine and culture are inseparable. In fact, some scholars (Payer, 1996; Lupton, 1994) have demonstrated that medicine is in fact as much a culture as it is science. A study of the British National Health Service (NHS) shows that the NHS is not just about healthcare, but is an integral part of the British culture (Hunter, 2008). The health system in a particular country reflects the health beliefs, illness behaviour, worldview, cultural values and level of development of that country (Lupton, 1994). Medicine does not exist in a vacuum. Medicine exists in a particular context. Healthcare, health policies and treatment decisions are all contextual issues (Hunter, 2008) and only make sense when studied in their particular context.

The practice of medicine differs from culture to culture (Freidson, 1970). In Britain, doctors do fewer tests and give less medicine and lower doses. Germans use six times the number of heart drugs as the French or English, although the three countries have similar rates of heart disease (Payer, 1996). France's medical community prefers to focus on the "terrain", or the vitality of the body, and choose gentle therapies such as natural medicines, nutritional supplements, and rest to strengthen and restore the terrain. When they do use pharmaceuticals, they prescribe lower dosages and shorter courses (five days instead of ten). This orientation toward shoring up the terrain has put French scientists and physicians in the lead in fields such as immunotherapy for cancer and AIDS.

In the United States of America, the emphasis is on aggressive treatments using high-tech equipment with special focus on surgical interventions. The American attitude is to view disease as a hostile invasion by foreign bodies, whether viruses or bacteria, and then declare war on the "invader". American doctors perform more diagnostic tests than doctors in France, Germany or Britain. They prefer invasive surgery to drug treatment, and when they use drugs, they are likely to use higher doses and more aggressive drugs. An American woman has two to three times the chance of having a hysterectomy (a surgical procedure to remove a woman's womb) as her counterpart in England, France or Germany. Over 60 percent of hysterectomies in the US are performed on women aged under forty-four. Many American doctors consider it routine to perform hysterectomies for women around the age of forty, especially if there is any slight pointer to cancer. In Nigeria, most women, even of menopausal age, would consider a hysterectomy as a very last resort, while some don't even consider it as an option at all, even under pain of death. Tampering with the womb for any reason is considered a taboo by many Nigerian women. A simplistic explanation would be to regard this perspective as religious naivety. But the matter is far too complex to be explained away by religion alone.

Medical practice is also influenced by the way doctors are remunerated in various countries. Since prices of medical procedures are fixed in advance, the only way a French doctor, for example, can increase his income is by performing more services. Therefore, if a French doctor wants to double his income, he takes out as many appendixes as possible, whereas if an American doctor wants to double his income, he doubles his fees (Lupton, 1994). American doctors whose insurance companies would require them to perform a caesarean section after fibroid removal are more likely to remove the uterus than French doctors who face no such pressure.

In Nigeria, the majority of doctors who work in government hospitals also have their own private clinics. This practice is outlawed in Europe and America as well as in Nigeria. The difference is that while this law is dutifully enforced in other countries, in Nigeria it exists only on paper. This has encouraged doctors to refer many of their patients to their own private clinics. The majority of non-complicated surgeries in Nigeria are therefore done in private clinics owned by government-employed doctors.

Different cultures place importance on different organs. The French place more attention on the liver, with its ability to process food and to regulate the body. The Germans focus on the heart. A beautiful woman in French culture has a slim body, is tall, and has straight, smooth legs, clear skin and medium-sized breasts. A beautiful American woman is expected to have large breasts. For the German, the heart is all that matters. In Eastern and Western Nigeria, being moderately fat is considered beautiful and attractive in a woman. Like Nigerians, the French value fertility and will do everything possible to preserve it. This explains why French doctors would use a hysterosalpingogram (an infertility test that shows whether both fallopian tubes are open and whether the shape of the uterine cavity is normal), because they are afraid of adhesions from surgery that might impair fertility, rather than the D&C (dilation and curettage) that German, English and Americans use to diagnose conditions.

As mentioned above, American doctors carry out excessive hysterectomies that would be considered unwarranted in England, France and Germany. And where French and German doctors would do lumpectomies (surgical excision of a tumour from the breast with the removal of a minimal amount of surrounding tissue), American doctors are likely to opt for radical mastectomies (surgical removal of one or both breasts).

It is not true that people choose traditional/alternative medicine because they are too poor to afford biomedicine (Dean, 2005). Some 39 percent of French doctors and 20 percent of German doctors prescribe alternative medicines. More than 40 percent of British general practitioners refer patients to alternative medicine practitioners, especially homeopathic doctors, and 45 percent of Dutch physicians consider alternative remedies effective. Recognizing that over 50 percent of its population is using homeopathy, herbal medicine and other natural healing therapies, Canada established the Office of Natural Health Products in March 1999. The right to choose one's preferred health system is as fundamental as the right to free speech, and must be respected by responsible governments.

"Overdosed America" is the title of a book by American medical practitioner John Abramson (2008), that laments how the profit motive has taken over healthcare in America, and of course the culture is fast spreading to other parts of the world, including Africa. Abramson observed that new "normals" are frequently adopted for blood pressure, cholesterol levels and blood sugar which are based more on market forces than on science, while new "diseases" like osteoporosis and erectile dysfunction have been developed. Too fat, too thin, too sad, too happy... whatever the problem is, biotech is developing a vaccine or a pill to cure us. The world we live in is a world where all our worries can be medicated away. Loss of a job, the death of a loved one or even a pet is often treated with antidepressants that are otherwise indicated for major depressive disorders. Biotech not only treats our diseases; it often invents diseases and then goes ahead and provides the medication to cure its inventions. The American Psychiatric Association will soon recognise being a "shopaholic" as a clinical disorder. At Stanford University, trials held on the SSRI anti-depressant Citalopram concluded that the drug was a safe and effective treatment for Compulsive Shopping Disorder.

In 2011, clinics to treat internet addiction opened in the US and China. What were once considered normal human events and common human problems pregnancy, birth, aging, menopause, alcoholism and obesity – are now viewed as medical conditions. For better or worse, medicine increasingly permeates aspects of daily life. Intense advertising by pharmaceutical companies ensure that patients put pressure on their doctors to prescribe drugs that are often useless. Science-based lifestyle changes are all too often under-utilised in patients at risk of heart disease, cancer, hypertension or diabetes, in favour of using medications as a first-line approach.

In the race to achieve the Millennium Development Goals, combat increasing drug resistance and tackle new diseases, traditional medicine is making a comeback. The World Health Organization's Beijing Declaration in 2008 marked a milestone in acknowledging the need to integrate traditional medicine into national health systems. Governments, drug companies, researchers and international aid organisations increasingly recognise the value of traditional medicine and its practitioners – both as a source of potential new blockbuster drugs and as alternative providers of primary healthcare. After years of ambivalence on the issue of traditional and alternative medicine, some African governments are now considering giving traditional medicine formal status in the national health system. This volte-face is a result of the dire needs their countries face in health care, the inability of the biomedical approach to meet these needs, and the alarming deadly side effects of supposedly "safe" drugs.

Some researchers have observed that the great improvement in health and wellbeing in the developed countries of Europe and America was not as a result of better medication, more hospitals or medical breakthroughs (Nijhawan, 2010; Mendelsohn, 1979; Dean, 2005). Rather, it was a result of disease-preventing habits such as improved hygiene, good drainage systems and good dietary habits. Evidence from surveys has shown that many prevalent diseases can be prevented and managed through proper health education, healthy dietary habits and physical exercise (World Bank, 2010). What Africa needs is not necessarily more hospitals, more sophisticated diagnostic equipment or more aggressive drugs. Rather, Africa needs more health educationists, more nutritionists, more health counsellors and more preventive health care specialists. Indeed, prevention is better than cure.

It is no accident that the golden age of modern medicine and drug discovery, from 1900 to 1950, was the period when science was not yet disconnected from nature, when scientists tilled the soil, refined their gifts for the observation of nature and the human body, and were in touch with the natural environment. After many years of wandering in the wilderness of genetic engineering, genetic screening and gene therapy, costing billions of dollars in research with little to show for it, modern science is now looking back toward the African bush. Could it be that the next blockbuster drug is lying somewhere there?

Many traditional healers in Africa have died and more continue to die without passing on their knowledge and expertise to their children or apprentices. The children often show no interest in taking over the healing work from their parents, but rather have migrated to the cities in search of white-collar jobs. Some became fiery evangelists, pastors and Christian fanatics who wage "war" on traditional medicine, which they regard as "pagan", "idolatrous" and "fetishist". As a result, much useful knowledge on healing plants and medicines is being lost – knowledge that appears worthless because it is not properly valued. This book is a contribution to efforts to preserve such indigenous knowledge, especially traditional medical knowledge in Africa. It is the fruit of over 15 years' research and fieldwork documenting the healing plants traditionally used for medicine in different parts of Nigeria, especially the southern part of Nigeria. In the belief system of the traditional healers, every plant has a reason for existing. Plants grow for a particular purpose. Every plant is a manifestation of the energy field which is the universe; a mirror reflecting the intensity and nature of the energy field of the particular environment where they grow. Some plants exist to give nourishment to the earth. Some exist to give support to other plants. Some grow to help regulate the exchange of oxygen and carbon dioxide between human beings and plants. Some give information about past, current and coming events: the coming of rain or a drought, or an epidemic. The types of plants growing in a particular place often reflect the need or problem in that place. Shortly before any epidemic or disease, the plant which has the antidote begins to sprout. A plant growing in a house of happy and fulfilled people is radiant, attractive and healthy, even when little attention is given to it. On arrival in a new place, experienced herbalists and mystics can gauge the prevalent sicknesses and mood simply by observing the kinds of plants growing nearby. For every disease or deficiency, there is always a medicinal plant growing nearby. It is up to human beings to open nature's book of Wisdom and learn how to use these plants.

There is a very close link between plants and animals: so close that several of the plants we know derive their names from this relationship. We have catnip, horsetail, goat weed, bird's eye, cat eye and pigweed, among many others. There are over 400,000 species of plants on this planet. Human beings in different continents use about 100,000 of these plants for medicinal purposes. Of these, only 10,000 are said to have been clinically analyzed and thus recommended for human consumption.

In traditional African communities, plants are believed to speak many languages. Do plants speak? The answer is yes. Plants speak. Animals speak. Human beings speak. Nature speaks. Intercommunication and interconnectivity is the nature of the universe. But what language do plants speak? Such a question reflects how limited we are in our understanding of reality. We often mistake speech for communication. But speech, the vocal sound we produce, is only one of the means of communication, and it is the most limited. In fact, only 30 per cent of our communication is done through speech. The rest is through gestures, facial expressions, and other forms of body language. Failure to always remember this has led to so much misunderstanding in our world. Plants are very sensitive to sound and can pick up sound vibrations long before they reach the human ear. The adult human ear can hear any sound that vibrates within the frequency of 20Hz to 20,000Hz, babies can detect sounds as high as 50,000Hz, while dogs and other animals can hear sounds with a frequency as high as 100,000Hz. Plants can detect sounds of over 100,000Hz frequencies.

There is so much in nature that is outside the range of our human perceptiveness and experience. The fact that we do not perceive something does not mean that it does not exist. It only shows how limited we are, and thus should make us humble. In the ancient Yoruba culture, the use of sound to create things was highly developed. Yoruba hunters, warriors and herbalists were believed to have a deep knowledge of sound mysteries. Wars were fought not with guns or knives, but with potent speech. The warring groups stood face to face and engaged each other in a war of chants. The side that was able to utter sounds that evoked higher vibratory frequency gained control over the other side, who would become weak and helpless and were then captured. It was believed that through the manipulation of sound, trees could be transformed into animals, water into blood, bad into good.

In African societies, the use of creative sound to affect matter came in the form of pronunciation of names. By uttering the name of a thing, one evokes a response in it. A number of plants and animals are particularly sensitive to sound, such as plants of the Jathroph species. Yoruba herbal mystics call Jathropha different names depending on what they want to use it for. When they want to use it to attend to a predominantly physical problem, they call it *Lapalapa*. When it is to treat a predominantly spiritual problem, they call it *Iyalode*. And when it is for both physical and spiritual treatment, they call it *Botuje*. By calling it a particular name, they control the vibratory radiation of the plant and condition it to work in the desired way (Adodo, 2003).

Another sound-sensitive plant is *Hypoestes verticillaris*, called Ogbo in Yoruba. Ogbo is used by African mystics and herbalists to cure insomnia, psychosis and cancer, and as an effective help for women in difficult labour. Ogbo is very effective in dissolving fibroid tumours. In fact, the use of Ogbo roots and leaves for treating fibroids is one of the hidden treasures of traditional herbal medicine, and is in urgent need of further rigorous scientific investigation.

In traditional African medicine, the shape and peculiarity of a plant is believed to be a reliable source of information about the nature of the plant. In many African societies, and indeed in other parts of the world, people look at the colour and shape as well as the location of a plant to get an insight into its use and importance. This is called the "Doctrine of signatures" and is based on the belief that plants grow in a specific area because there is a need for them. Herbs that grow on mountains are believed to be good for the respiratory system – lungs, bronchi, nostrils and the nervous system. They are said to cure high blood pressure as well as pneumonia. Herbs that grow in water are regarded as very medicinal and are almost always edible, since poisonous herbs very rarely grow in water. They are believed to be good for the circulatory system and to help in repairing the liver and kidneys. Herbs that grow in water are also believed to be good for treating all forms of infertility in both men and women. Herbs that grow close to the soil are believed to be good for digestive and circulatory problems. Since they are close to the ground, the mineral content is high, and so they are thought to be good for the bones and blood. Those who suffer from anaemia would find these herbs useful (Engel, 2002). Of course, the doctrine of signatures does not hold true in all cases, but that is not a reason to condemn the whole theory.

From time to time, traditional healers prescribe that certain herbs be harvested only at a particular time of the day. Sometimes they insist that certain plants should be harvested before sunrise, some after sunset. At times they go out themselves in the middle of the night to collect particular herbs. This practice in itself is scientifically correct. During the night, the chemical compounds in many plants, especially trees, settle down to the roots. Therefore, in order to get the best out of these roots, it is advisable to harvest them at sunset, which in tropical countries begins from 5pm.

When the sun begins to rise, plants (especially trees) draw up their chemical compounds and distribute them to the leaves and bark. By the middle of the day, these compounds are fully concentrated in the leaves.

For this reason, the best time to harvest the leaves of medicinal plants is at midday, when the sun is about to reach its peak. By late afternoon, the chemical compounds in trees begin their downward journey back to the roots through the stems and barks. For this reason, the best time to collect the bark of a tree is late in the afternoon or in the early evening, before sunset. Now, somebody may come and tell you to do your harvesting at 10pm rather than 5pm. They may tell you that the roots will not work for you unless you harvest them at 10 or 11pm or at midnight. The background of our scientific knowledge tells us that this extra detail or explanation is untrue or unnecessary; however, the basic idea of harvesting the root at sunset is well founded. A traditional healer may colour this common-sense science with riddles and rituals simply to increase the mystery surrounding his practice and to preserve his prestige.

It is not the will of God that we throw away the wisdom of our forefathers and mothers. The challenge for today's African thinkers, scientists and philosophers is to sift out the fetish and superstitions from our inherited deposits of knowledge without throwing away the truth. This book sets an example of how this could be done, and explains why it should be done.

References

Abramson, J. (2008) 'Overdosed America: The Broken Promise of American Medicine'. New York: Harper Perennial

Adodo, A. (2003) 'The Healing Radiance of the Soul'. Lagos: Agelex

Adodo, A. (2011) 'Disease and Dietary Patterns in Edo Central Nigeria: An Epidemiological Survey': Saarbrücken: Lambert Academic Publishing

Adodo, A. (2017) 'Integral Community Enterprise in Africa Communitalism as an Alternative to Capitalism'. London: Routledge.

Dean, C. (2005) 'Death by Modern Medicine'. USA: Matrix Verite.

Engel, C. (2002) 'Wild Health: How Animals Keep Themselves Well and What we can Learn from Them'. Boston: Houghton Mifflin Harcourt

Freidson E. (1970) 'Professional Dominance: The Social Structure of Medical Care'. New York: Atherton Press.

Hunter, D. (2008) 'The health debate'. Bristol, UK: The Policy Press.

Le Grand, A. and Wondergem, P. (1990) 'Herbal medicine and health promotion'. Amsterdam: Royal Tropical Institute.

Lupton, D. (1994) 'Medicine as Culture'. London: Sage Publications.

Mendelsohn, R. (1979) 'Confessions of a Medical Heretic'. New York: McGraw Hill.

Nijhawan, N. (2010) 'Modern Medicine is Killing You'. Washington Ave.: L.E.O Publishing.

Payer, L. (1996) 'Medicine and Culture'. New York: Henry Holt.

World Bank working paper No. 187 (2010) 'Improving Primary Health Care Delivery in Nigeria. Evidence from Four States'. Washington DC: AHD series.

Chapter 1

The Practice of
Medicine in Africa

Africa is home to diverse and innumerable tribes, ethnic and social groups. Some represent huge populations consisting of millions of people, while others are smaller groups of a few thousand. Some countries have over 100 different ethnic groups (for example Nigeria, with over 250 ethnic groups) with varied culturally based values and belief systems.

In all African societies during the early epoch, the individual at every stage of life had a series of duties and obligations to others in the society, as well as a set of rights: namely, things that he or she could expect or demand from other individuals. Age and sex were the most important factor determining the extent of a person's rights and obligations. The oldest members of the society were highly respected and usually in positions of authority, and the idea of seniority through age was reflected in the presence of age-graded groups in a great many African societies.

Plants have formed the basis of sophisticated traditional medicine practices that have been used for thousands of years by people in China, India, Nigeria and many other countries (Farnsworth and Soejarto, 1991). Perhaps as early as Neanderthal man, plants were believed to have healing power (WHO, 1978b). The earliest records of civilisation from the ancient cultures of Africa, China, Egypt and the Indus valley reveal evidence in support of the use of herbal medicine (Baqar, 2001). These include the Atharva Veda, which is the basis for Ayurvedic medicine in India (dating back to 2000 BCE), the clay tablets in Mesopotamia (1700 BCE), and the Eber Papyrus in Egypt (1550 BCE) (Kumar et al., 1997). Other famous literature sources on medicinal plants include "De materia medica" written by Dioscorides between CE 60 and 78, and Jing's classic of Chinese traditional medicine, the "Divine Farmer's Materia Medica" (written around 200 CE) (Joy et al., 1998).

History and practice of traditional African medicine

As with food technology, Africans had evolved their medical technology long before colonialism. According to Andah (1992), from very early times, Africans used plants as curatives and palliatives for various ailments. Successful treatments became formalised, sometimes with prescriptions outlining the correct methods of preparation and dosage. Andah stated that in many cases, patients were cured of their physical or psychological ailments. African traditional medicine is ancient, and is perhaps the most diverse of all medicinal systems. Africa is considered to be the cradle of humankind, with a rich biological and cultural diversity, and marked regional differences in healing practices. African traditional medicine in its varied forms is holistic, involving both the body and the mind. The healer typically diagnoses and treats the psychological basis of an illness before prescribing medicines to treat the symptoms.

Generally speaking, the methods applied by African traditional healers are similar across the continent, although the plants used and the therapeutic values attributed to them are dependent on various factors. Some of these factors are geographical, sociological and economic, and transcend ethnic, national and political boundaries.

According to Onu (1999), indigenous medical technology in Africa has not only developed drugs and surgical skills for fighting ailments but is founded on a rational and coherent body of knowledge, which can be used to train specialists in the healing of various diseases and disorders. Traditional medical practice in Africa developed since antiquity to the stage of setting bones, healing mental disorders and even conducting relatively complicated operations such as caesarean sections. A picture of indigenous medical practice in Africa is, therefore, a picture of specialists trained in the acquisition of an impressive wealth of knowledge around herbs and other materials of therapeutic value. Through inspiration, observation and experiments involving trial and error, the medical value of the plant kingdom, minerals and certain animals was gradually realised and exploited.

Plant-based medicine is so prominent in Africa that a distinct class of practitioners has emerged with a thorough knowledge of the medicinal properties of plants and the pharmaceutical steps necessary to turn them into drugs. In addition to herbal materials, minerals such as clay, salt, stone and many other substances have been used as raw ingredients in indigenous pharmaceutical practice. Ubrurhe (2003) drew attention to the lzon ethnic group of the Niger Delta in Nigeria, whose environment does not permit the growth of many herbs and who, as an alternative, specialise in massage. According to Ubrurhe, this therapeutic system has been employed for the treatment of ailments of the nervous, muscular and osseous systems as well as for treating gynaecological problems. The armamentarium of the masseur is the physical manipulation of the muscles, joints and veins through the bare skin. In most cases, massage treatment may be applied to relax the muscles and veins as well as to improve circulation of blood. Ubrurhe concluded that this therapeutic method has spread to the lzon's neighbours – the Urhobo, lsoko and Itsekiri.

Writing on hydrotherapy, Ubrurhe (2003) contended that its curative value is realised by both the practitioner and those who have undergone such treatment, and more recently by scientists. By equalizing the circulation of the blood in all the systems of the body, hydrotherapy helps to increase muscular tone and nerve force, improving nutrition and digestion, and thereby increasing the activity of the respiratory glands. Hydrotherapy facilitates the elimination of broken-down tissue cells and poisonous matters. It involves the use of cold, hot, compressed and steamed vapour baths. Herbs which are added to cold or hot baths are used for the treatment of different diseases and ailments including fever, headache, rheumatism and general pains. The hot bath not only makes the skin capillaries relax but also increases the activity of the sweat glands. It has been observed that water increases the absorption of oxygen to about 75%, while about 85% of the carbon dioxide in the body is eliminated through the use and consumption of water. Ubrurhe (2003) also wrote extensively on the practice of "cupping" or blood-letting as a therapy – the method of abstracting impure blood using abstraction cups or horns. He asserted that this is widely practised in Africa, especially in Northern Nigeria, where it has been regarded as an effective treatment for rheumatism and morbid conditions of the blood. Traditional medical practitioners in Africa are adept in performing intricate surgical operations to remove bullets and poisonous arrows from wounded traditional fighters, extricating infected tissues and stitching the wound together, then applying calabash to promote healing. Traditional plants with anaesthetic properties are applied to remove or reduce pain before the operation.

Sofowora (1982) observed that in traditional medicine, burns are treated with herbal preparations which produce a soothing effect. For example, in cases of superficial burns, ointments prepared from papaya juice are applied by Ayurveda practitioners to gradually remove dead tissue. When this process is complete, and the healthy granulation tissue appears, the burn is treated with a herbal medication specially prepared to promote healing. Sofowora (1982) further observed that bone-setting is a specialised area of traditional medicine. It is usually performed without the aid of X-rays; the experienced traditional bone-setter uses his hands and fingers to feel and assess the type and extent of damage to a broken bone. In the case of a broken leg, the patient is made to lie or sit down with the fractured leg lying flat. Herbal dressings are placed on the fracture before planks or sticks are tied around the leg using string or the stem of a climbing plant.

Many traditional medical practitioners have a diverse range of skills and abilities: they may also be psychotherapists and proficient in faith healing (spiritual healing), apiutic occultism, male and female circumcision, making tribal marks, treating snakebites and whitlow, removing tuberculosis lymphadenitis in the neck, cutting the umbilical cord, piercing earlobes, removing the uvula (uvulectomy), extracting decayed teeth, trephination (drilling a hole in the skull, also known as trepanation), abdominal surgery, preventive medicine and so on. As far back as 1884, Dr. R.W. Felkin observed a caesarean section among the Bunyoro people of Uganda. Imperato (1977) reported that the patient was first narcotised with herbal preparations. The bleeding vessels were cauterised with red-hot iron rods. Blood was then drained from the abdominal cavity before the uterus was cut open and the baby and placenta carefully removed. The incision in the uterus was then sutured using iron spikes and string made from tree bark. The wound was then covered with herbal pastes, a hot banana leaf and finally a cloth bandage.

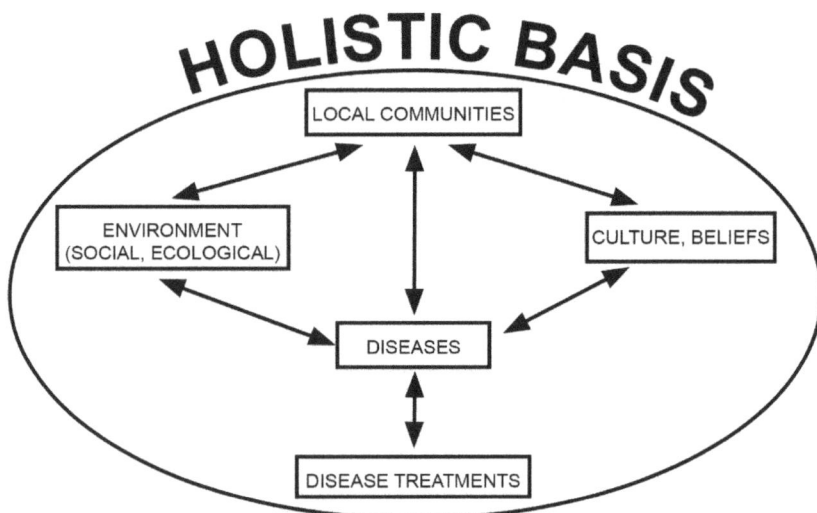

HOLISTIC BASIS

```
                    LOCAL COMMUNITIES

ENVIRONMENT                                  CULTURE, BELIEFS
(SOCIAL, ECOLOGICAL)

                    DISEASES

                    DISEASE TREATMENTS
```

In traditional African healers' understanding, the healing process is holistic (Thorpe, 1993). This implies that the healer deals with the whole person and provides treatment for physical, psychological, spiritual and social symptoms. Traditional healers do not separate the natural from the spiritual, or the physical from the supernatural. This means they address health issues from two major perspectives—physical and spiritual.

1. **Physical perspective:** The following are some of the healing processes used when the sickness is deemed to have physical causes:

a. *Prescription of herbs:* The traditional healer may prescribe herbs, depending on the kind of disease the patient has presented with. These prescriptions come with specific instructions on how to prepare the herb, the dose and timeframe for use (Ayim-Aboagye, 1993, Lartey, 1986).

b. *Application of clay and herbs:* In some cases, the traditional healer prepares white clay with herbs for the patient to apply on his or her body for a number of days; this is used particularly in the case of skin diseases. This concept is based on the spiritual belief that the human body is made from dust or the earth, so in order to heal it you to return to where it came from. Clay and particular herbs are also sometimes used in preventive rituals, to prevent the spirits behind the illness from attacking the patient (White, 2015).

c. *Counselling:* Sometimes the patient is advised on how to live his or her life, especially regarding the kind of food they should or should not eat. This is particularly the case when a taboo has been violated. The patient is advised to demonstrate good behaviour should it be felt that the disease occurred as a result of poor behaviour (Sundermeier, 1998).

2. **Spiritual/non-physical perspective:** When the cause of sickness is believed to be more than physical, or is thought to arise from a spiritual problem, the patient is encouraged to seek spiritual counselling and to carry out prayer and other rituals. Some of the healing processes used when the sickness is deemed to have spiritual causes are outlined below.

a. *Spiritual protection:* If the traditional healer perceives the disease to have been caused by an attack by evil spirits, the sufferer may be protected by the use of a talisman, charm, body marks made using "moto" (spiritually prepared black powder), amulets, or a "spiritual bath" to drive the evil spirits away (see "spiritual cleansing", below). These are rites aimed at eliminating evils or dangers that are seen to have taken root in a family or community (Westerlund, 2006).

b. *Sacrifices:* Sacrifices are sometimes offered at the perceived request of the spirits, gods and ancestors. Sometimes animals are slaughtered or buried alive (Olupona, 2004). Among the Ewes and some other tribes in northern Ghana, dogs or cats are sometimes buried alive at midnight to save the soul of a person at the point of death. It is believed that because dogs and cats are domestic animals, if someone very close to them is about to die, the animal can offer its life so that the person can live. So when a dog or cat dies mysteriously it is often interpreted that they have saved the life of a human. Animal sacrifices are also carried out in some societies as part of spiritual cleansing (see below).

c. *Spiritual cleansing:* In some cases, herbs are prepared for the patient to bathe with at particular times of day for a number of days. Sometimes an animal is slaughtered and the blood poured on the head and feet of the patient as a way of cleansing. This practice is also common among the Ewe communities in Ghana (Westerlund, 2006).

d. *Appeasing the gods:* According to interviews with some traditional priests (diviners) in Kumasi in the Ashanti region of Ghana, if diseases are seen to have been caused by the invocation of a curse or a violation of taboos, the diviner appeases the ancestors, spirits or gods. This is done according to the severity of the case, either by sacrificing an animal or by pouring of libation. In many cases, the affected person would be told to buy the ritual articles needed for the process, such as "spotless" animals (doves, cats, dogs, goats and fowl), liquor including schnapps or the traditional akpeteshie, calico (red, white or black), eggs or cola nuts. Following the rituals, the articles used are sometimes left at a particular place to rot, thrown into a river as required by the gods or spirits, or placed at a four-way junction or in the outskirts of the community, depending on the purpose of the ritual.

Exorcism: This is the practice of expelling demons or evil spirits from people or places that are believed to possessed. Exorcism is usually performed by a person with religious authority, such as a priest or shaman; it was common in ancient societies and was based on the practice of magic. In the ancient Babylonian civilisation, in what is now Iraq, special priests would destroy a clay or wax image of a demon in a ritual meant to destroy the actual demon. The ancient Egyptians and Greeks had similar rites, and many religions in various parts of the world continue the practice of exorcism (Encarta, 2009). For example, it is practised by the Ewes and some Akan tribes in Ghana, where exorcism is mostly carried out by singing, drumming, dancing, spraying powder into the air and onto the body of the possessed, or by striking their body serveral times with an animal tail until the spirit has been released. During the process, the possessed person rolls and struggles on the ground but becomes stable after the exorcism, usually with a deep sense of relief (White, 2015). Many traditional communities in Ghana are of the view that mental illness is mostly caused by evil spirits and requires exorcism. This approach is common practice, for example, in the Tigari shrines in Ghana.

Types of healers in African traditional health care

The traditional healer, as defined by the WHO (1976), is a person who is recognised by the community in which he or she lives as competent to provide health care using plant, animal and mineral substances and certain other methods based on the social, cultural and religious background, as well as on the knowledge, attributes and beliefs that are prevalent in the community regarding physical, mental and social wellbeing and the causation of disease and disability. The different types of healers in traditional African society are outlined below:

Traditional herbalists: Herbalists mainly use medicinal plants or parts of such plants including the whole root, stem, leaves, stem bark or root bark, flowers, fruits and seeds. Sometimes they also use animal parts or entire small animals (such as snails, snakes, chameleons, tortoises, lizards, etc.), as well as inorganic residues (including alum, camphor, salt, etc.) and insects (bees, black ants, etc.). Herbal preparations may be offered in the form of (i) a powder which can be swallowed or taken with pap (cold or hot) or any drink; (ii) a powder which is rubbed into incisions made on part of the body with a sharp knife; (iii) a preparation soaked in water or local gin, and decanted as required before drinking (the materials could alternatively be boiled in water, then cooled and strained); (iv) a preparation pounded with native soap and used for bathing—such medicated soaps are commonly used for skin diseases; (v) a paste, pomade or ointment in a medium of palm oil or shea butter; or (vi) a soup which is eaten by the patient.

The herbalist cures mainly with plants which he gathers fresh. When seasonal plants have to be used, these are collected when available and preserved, usually by drying (Ekeopara et al., 2017). Unlike the bone-setter, the traditional psychiatrist and the traditional birth attendant, whose duties are well defined and specialised (see below), the herbalist is the general practitioner of traditional medicine. He is expected to be knowledgeable in the various aspects of healing and in the functioning of all the organs of the body. By his wealth of experience and knowledge, he is expected to determine the nature of the patient's illness, treat him and also predict the course of his treatment. In a typical traditional setting, the herbalist combines the role of the present-day doctor with that of the pharmacist and the nurse (Ekeopara et al., 2017).

Traditional birth attendants: The WHO 1976 defines a traditional birth attendant (TBA) as a person who assists a mother in childbirth and who initially acquired her skills alone or working with other birth attendants. TBAs are usually older, experienced women who primarily see their role as contributing their skills for the good of the community. In northern Nigeria, TBAs are all women, whereas in some other parts of the country both males and females take on this role. TBAs occupy a prominent position in Nigeria today, particularly in rural areas; 60-85 percent of births in the country are assisted by TBAs (Ekeopara et al., 2017). TBAs can diagnose and confirm pregnancy, and determine the position of the growing foetus. They provide prenatal and postnatal care, thereby successfully combining the duties of the modern-day midwife.

As a result of their wide exposure and experience, many TBAs have been trained to assist in orthodox medical practices at the primary health care level, leading to a reduction in maternal and child mortality and morbidity (Ekeopara et al., 2017). Highly experienced TBAs have also been known to assist in obstetric and paediatric care, managing simple maternal and childhood illnesses. With experienced TBAs, delivery by caesarean section is uncommon, as it is not usually necessary to seek surgical help.

1. *Traditional surgeons:* The various forms of surgery recognised in traditional medical care include: (i) the cutting of tribal marks – traditional surgeons cut tribal marks into cheeks, bellies, etc. and rub charred herbal products into the wound to encourage the formation of scar tissue; (ii) male and female circumcision (clitoridectomy) – traditional surgeons carry out these simple surgical operations with special knives and scissors, and treat resulting bleeding and wounds with snail body fluid or pastes prepared from plants (these practices are, however, fast dying out in urban areas); and (iii) removal of whitlow – diseased toes or fingers are usually cut open and treated. Other forms of surgery include piercing of earlobes, particularly in young people, to allow the fixing of earrings; and extracting infected teeth before treating gums with herbal medicines prepared in local gin (Ekeopara et al., 2017).

2. *Traditional medicinal ingredient dealers:* These dealers, usually women, are involved in buying and selling the plants, animals, insects and minerals used in herbal preparations. Some dealers are also involved in preparing herbal concoctions or decoctions (herbal preparations created by boiling herbs in liquid, usually water) for managing or curing febrile conditions in children, or to treat other diseases in women and children; as such they may qualify to be referred to as traditional healers (Ekeopara et al., 2017).

3. *Traditional psychiatrists:* The traditional psychiatrist specialises in the treatment of mental disorders. People suffering violent forms of psychosis are restrained using iron chains or wooden shackles. Those who are regarded as being possessed by demons may be called or beaten into submission, and then given herbal hypnotics or highly sedative herbal potions to bring them to a state of mental, emotional and psychological calm. The treatment and rehabilitation of people with mental disorders usually takes place over a long period.

4. *Practitioners of therapeutic spiritism:* These include diviners or fortune tellers, who may be called "seers", "alfas" and "priests". They may use

supernatural or mysterious forces; prayers, chanting and singing of incantations, invocations or rituals associated with the community's religious worship; or prepare sacrificial materials to appease unknown gods. Practitioners are usually consulted on the diagnosis of diseases, their causes and treatment. With their perceived ability to deal with the unseen and the supernatural, they are usually held in high esteem in the community. They are believed to have extra-sensory perception, to be able to receive telepathic messages and consult oracles, spirit guides etc., and to perform well where other traditional healers and orthodox doctors fail.

It is believed that diseases which are caused by supernatural forces can be readily diagnosed and treated by these practitioners, and that certain medical ingredients have spiritual powers and can be effectively utilised by these practitioners for the good of all. These include ingredients from unusually large trees that are believed to house spirits; plants commonly found in graveyards, like the physic nut; protective plants, such as the wild colocynth or "Sodom apple"; or even some reproductive herbs, like the "sausage tree".

Some practitioners read and interpret the sounds made by "magic stones" when they are thrown to the ground. Some read messages in a pool or a glass of water. Others use the throwing of cowries, coins, kola-nut seeds, divining rods, keys or sticks, etc. (Ekeopara et al., 2017). Diviners seek input from the spiritual world to understand the cause of the illness and prescribe a cure (Asamoah-Gyadu, 2014 Cheetham and Griffiths, 1982). They are understood to play an intermediary role between the spirit world and the physical world; thus in some cultures they are called "the eyes of the spirits". According to Sundermeier (1998), diviners are believed to be the custodians of theories of healing, and the hope of society. They learn how to cause, cure and prevent disease, misfortune, infertility, poor crop yields magic, witchcraft and society.

The rise of allopathic medicine in Nigeria

Allopathic medicine, which is also referred to as "orthodox", "Western" or "conventional" medicine, is defined as medicine based on scientific methods and taught in Western medical schools (CSRC, 2005). Recorded European entry into Nigeria began when Portuguese explorers traded with the Benin Empire in 1472; traces of the influence of the Roman Catholic Church also date back to this time, and images of Portuguese soldiers abound in Benin bronzes. The Portuguese were credited with being the first people to bring Western medical care to their traders in outposts, but not to the indigenous African population (Schram, 1966). As the trade in human cargo expanded and accelerated, the high rate of infection with locally endemic diseases to which the previously unexposed European slave traders were subjected – notably malaria, yellow fever and the ubiquitous dysenteric diarrhoea – compelled the proprietors of the slave trade to introduce limited medical facilities for their staff. Throughout the period, healthcare facilities were available only on board the slave ships.

The first practising doctors of allopathic medicine in Nigeria were the medical missionaries, ship surgeons, medically qualified botanists and explorers who sailed into many ports and navigated several large rivers from the 17th century onwards. No hospitals were built on the mainland until the later part of 19th century, but there were hospitals in offshore islands three centuries earlier. In the mid-19th century, Dr. Williams, a Briton, was credited with carrying out several vaccination sessions and wound-dressing for indigenous populations along the West coast of Africa, including the Niger Delta and up to Lokoja (Schram, 1966). However, orthodox medicine was not formally introduced in Nigeria until the 1860s. The first group of Roman Catholic nuns in Nigeria lived in a convent in Lagos; later, led by Sister Maria of The Assumption, they moved to Abeokuta and worked under Father Francois, founder of the first full-fledged mainland hospital, the famous Sacred Heart Hospital, in Abeokuta (HERFON, 2006). This was followed by the British colonial government providing formal medical services, with the construction of hospitals and clinics in Lagos, Calabar and other coastal trading centres. Following this, a makeshift temporary civil hospital was built in Asaba (now in Delta State) in 1888. A government hospital was also built in Calabar in 1898, as a result of the wide impact of the first hospitals on the indigenous population and the colonial personnel and their families (HERFON, 2006). The role of the Christian missionaries in providing medical and health care services cannot be overemphasised. Reverend Hope Waddell, an Irish missionary of the United Presbyterian Church of Scotland (UPCS), worked for 30 years in the Calabar area, where he conducted Nigeria's first vaccination against smallpox; many of his missionary colleagues acquired skills and training that enabled them to run clinics and dispensaries in and around Calabar (HERFON, 2006).

Henry Townsend and David Hinderer founded the Church Missionary Society (CMS) (Yoruba Mission) and oversaw the mission's activities in Lagosand Abeokuta. In 1864, the Churchof England consecrated Reverend Samuel Ajayi Crowther as the Bishop of Western Equatorial Africa. He undertook a mission up the Niger as far as Lokoja, and from there to Calabar by the way of the Cross River and into South Cameroon. The establishment of various healthcare posts followed in the wake of Crowther's Episcopal missions. The Qua Iboe Mission, founded in 1891, established a number of dispensary and maternity services in southern Nigeria, as did the Baptist Mission. One of the most outstanding legacies of the Baptist Mission is the famous Baptist Hospital in Ogbomosho. A coalition of the protestant missions built the reputed Iyi Enu Hospital near Onitsha in 1906. The Sudan Interior Mission (SIM), founded in 1893, worked in the core of Nigeria and the predominantly Islamic north. It operated in the early days with two medical stations, in Bida and Pategi (HERFON, 2006).

The religious missions also contributed substantially to the training of nurses and paramedical personnel. A good example is the highly reputed nursing school of the SIM Christian Hospital in Vom. The mission hospitals in Shaki, Ogbomosho, Ilesa and Eku among others performed similarly important health-training roles. The missions also sponsored many of the first-generation Nigerian doctors to undertake professional training in Europe (HERFON, 2006). During the First World War of 1914–1918, substantial numbers of European health care personnel were withdrawn from Nigeria to render professional services for war victims. The Army Medical Corps (AMC) was set up by Lord Lugard in Lokoja, and was the forerunner of government medical services in Nigeria. It was a centralised medical service, which was initially military and later colonial in nature. In 1943, British colonials opened the first orthopaedic centre in Igbobi, Lagos, as a rehabilitation camp for wounded soldiers returning to Nigeria from the Second World War. The Yaba Medical School (YMS) was founded in 1930 to train a cadre of medical assistants, but ceased to exist after the establishment of University College Hospital, Ibadan. The Kano Medical School was inaugurated in 1954. From the 1500s, medical knowledge passed with enslaved Africans to the Americas for many centuries. Indeed, smallpox inoculation was introduced to North America by an enslaved African medical pioneer called Onesimus.

Allopathic medicine and African traditional medicine: a clash of world views

The impact of colonialism in Africa is characterised in ways that range from "fortune" to "agony". Some scholars (such as Curtin, 1989) are of the opinion that the process of modernisation in Africa is intrinsically connected with foreign intervention, particularly in areas of health and democracy. Curtin (1998) argues that the period between 1840 and 1860 was marked by significant and rapid innovation in tropical medicine, notably the invention of quinine to stem the scourge of malaria in the most endemic region of the world. From this perspective, the institutionalisation of the modern health care system is seen as one of many positive "legacies" of Western encroachment in Africa.

On the contrary, there are those who believe that Western "invasion" was/ is a setback in the process of development in Africa (Achebe, 1958; Afisi, 2009) particularly in modes of knowledge production (Taiwo, 1993). These scholars mention slavery, capitalism, colonialism and imperialism, neo-colonialism, and all forms of domination and exploitation that were embedded in these epochs, as major stumbling blocks to indigenous African development. Indeed, the current political and socio-economic crises in Africa are often attributed to colonialism. While some critics of colonialism have focused on its economic and political impacts, others have shifted attention to the impact of colonialism on the indigenous knowledge system (Mapara, 2009), and especially knowledge of medicine (Feierman, 2002; Konadu, 2008; Millar, 2004; Paul, 1977). Such arguments underscore the negative impact of colonialism on indigenous medicine. It is explained that the introduction of Western medicine and culture gave rise to a cultural-ideological clash that undermined and stigmatised the traditional health care system in Africa. In some extreme cases, traditional medicine was banned outright; for instance, the South African Medical Association outlawed the traditional medical system in South Africa in 1953 (Hassimet al. n.d). In addition, the Witchcraft Suppression Act of 1957 and the Witchcraft Suppression Amendment Act of 1970 declared traditional medicine unconstitutional, thereby prohibiting practitioners in South Africa (Hassim et al. n.d.).

The banning of traditional medicine was partially based on the belief that the concept of disease and illness in Africa was historically embedded in "witchcraft"; a perception which, in Western knowledge, reinforces negative ideas of "backwardness", "superstition" and of Africa as "the dark continent". However, as this book describes and as recent studies have shown, etiologies of illnesses in Africa are viewed from both natural and supernatural perspectives (Bello, 2006; Erinosho, 1998, 2005, 2006; Jegede, 1996; Oke, 1995). The subjugation of traditional medicine continued in most African countries even after independence, although local efforts were initiated to challenge the condemnation and stigmatisation of traditional medicine in some African communities during and after colonialism. Erinosho (1998, 2006) reported that the first protest against the marginalisation of traditional medicine in Nigeria dates back to 1922, when a group of native healers insisted that their medicine be legally recognised.

Onu (1999) stressed that drugless therapy is the area of African medical practice which has been most misunderstood. He noted that with the characteristic hypocrisy that goes with such misunderstanding, African traditional medicine has been regarded not only as ineffective, but as a primitive phenomenon, flourishing on ignorance and prelogical thinking—a misunderstanding that persists, even in enlightened circles. Onu (1999) concluded that it persists because of two unresolved issues in traditional medical practice: first, the controversy over the causes of diseases; and second, the fact that indigenous medical practice in Africa is yet to articulate meticulous models for explaining many sensitive aspects of its drugless therapy.

References

Achebe, C. (1958) 'Things Fall Apart'. UK: Heinemann Books Ltd.

Afisi, O.T. (2009) 'Tracing Contemporary Africa's Conflict Situation to Colonialism: A Breakdown of Communication among Natives'. Philosophical Papers and Reviews, 1(4): 59–66.

Andah, B.W. (1992) 'Nigeria's Indigenous Technology'. Ibadan: Ibadan University Press.

Asamoah-Gyadu, J.K. (2014) 'Therapeutic strategies in African religions: Health, herbal medicines and indigenous Christian spirituality'. Studies in World Christianity 20(1), 83. http://dx.doi.org/10.3366/swc.2014.0072.

Ayim-Aboagye, D. (1993) 'The function of myth in Akan healing experience: A psychological inquiry into two traditional Akan healing communities', PhD thesis, Dept. of Theology, Uppsala University.

Baqar, S.R. (2001) 'Anti-Spasmodic Action of Crude Methanolic Extract'. Journal of Medical Plants Res.Vol. 6(3) 461–464.

Bello, R.A. (2006) 'Integrating the Traditional and Modern Health Care System in Nigeria: A Policy Option for Better Access to Health Care Delivery'. In H. Saliu, A. Jimoh and T. Arosanyin (eds.), The National Question and Some Selected Topical Issues on Nigeria. Ibadan: Vantage Publishers.

Center for the Study of Religion and Culture (CSRC) (2005). 'Use of traditional vs. orthodox medicine in help-seeking behavior for psychiatric disorders in Nigeria'. Summer Fellowship Report 2005.

Cheetham, R.W.S. and Griffiths J.A. (1982) 'The traditional healer/ diviner as psychotherapist', South African Medical Journal 62, 957–958.

Curtin, P.D. (1989) 'Death by Migration: Europe's Encounter with the Tropical World in the Eighteenth Century'. London: Cambridge University Press.

Curtin, P.D. (1998). 'Disease and Empire: The Health of European Troops in theConquest of Africa'. London: Cambridge University Press.

Ekeopara, Chike Augustine, Ugoha, Azubuike M.I. (2017) 'The Contributions of African Traditional Medicine to Nigeria's Health Care Delivery System'. IOSR Journal of Humanities and Social Science (IOSR- JHSS) Volume 22, Issue 5, Ver. 4 (May 2017) pp. 32–43 e-ISSN: 2279-0837, p-ISSN: 2279-0845.

Encarta (2009) 'Exorcism', Microsoft® Student [DVD], Redmond. Erinosho et al. (1985) 'Traditional Medicine in Nigeria: A Study Prepared for the Federal Ministry of Health', Lagos, Nigeria.

Erinosho, O.A. (1998) 'Health Sociology for Universities, Colleges and Health Related Institutions'. Ibadan: Sam Bookman.

Erinosho, O.A. (2005) 'Sociology for Medical, Nursing, and Allied Professions inNigeria'. Abuja: Bulwark Consult.

Erinosho, O.A. (2006) 'Health Sociology for Universities, Colleges and Health Related Institutions'. Ibadan: Abuja: Bulwark Consult. Reprint

Farnsworth, N.R. and Soejarto, D.D. (1991) 'Global Importance of Medical Plants'. In Akerele, O., Heywood, V. and Synge, H. (Eds) Conservation of Medical Plants, pp. 200–250. Cambridge: Cambridge University Press.

Feierman, S. (2002) 'Traditional Medicine in Africa: Colonial Transformations'. NewYorkAcademy of Medicine. 13 March. Reported by Carter, G.M. Foundation for Integrative AIDS Research.

Hassim, A., Heywood, M. and Berger, J. (n.d.) 'Health and Democracy' (accessed at http://www.alp.org.za on 12January2010).

HERFON Nigerian Health Review (2006) Publication of Health Reform Foundation of Nigeria.

Imperato, P.J. (1977) 'African Folk Medicine: Practices and Beliefs of the Bambara and other People'. New York: Baltimore.

Jegede, A.S. (1996) 'Social Epidemiology'. In E.A. Oke and B.E. Owumi (eds.) Readingsin Medical Sociology. Ibadan: Resource Development and Management Services(RDMS).

Joy, P.P., Thomas, J., Mathew, S. and Skaria, B.P. (1998) 'Medical Plants'. Kerala Agricultural University, Aromatic and Medicinal Plant Research Station.

Mapara, J. (2009) 'Indigenous Knowledge Systems in Zimbabwe: Juxtaposing Postcolonial Theory'. The Journal of Pan African Studies, 3(1): 139–155.

Millar, D. (2004) 'Interfacing Two Knowledge Systems: Local Knowledge and Sciencein Africa'. Paper for the Compas Panel in the Conference: Bridging Scales and Epistemologies: Linking Local Knowledge with Global Science in Multi-Scale Assessments. Alexandria March.

Oke, E.A. (1995) 'Traditional Health Services: An Investigation of Providers and the Level and Pattern of Utilization among the Yoruba'. Ibadan Sociological Series, No. 1: 2–5.

Olupona, J.K. (2004) 'Owner of the day and regulator of the universe: Ifa Divination and healing among the Yoruba of South-Western Nigeria' in M. Winkelman and P.M. Peeks (eds.) Divination and healing: Potent vision, pp.103–117. Tucson, AZ: University of Arizona Press.

Onu, A.O. (1999) 'Social Basis of Illness: A Search for Therapeutic Meaning' in Okpoko, A.I. (ed). Africa's Indigenous Technology. Ibadan: Wisdom Publishers Ltd.

Paul, J. (1977) 'Medicine and Imperialism in Morocco'. MERIP Reports, 60: 3–12. 49.

Sarpong, K.P. (2002) 'People differ: An approach to inculturation in evangelism'. Accra: Sub-Sahara Publishers.'

Schram, R. (1966) 'Development of Nigerian Health services, 1940– 1960'. MD Thesis accepted by the Cambridge University, UK, under the title 'A brief history of public health in Nigeria', 1966. Published by the University of Ibadan Press in 1971 under the title, 'A History of the Nigerian Health Services'.

Sofowora, A. (1982) 'Medicinal Plants and Traditional Medicine in Africa'. Ibadan: Spectrum Books

Sundermeier, T. (1998) 'The individual and community in African traditional religions'. Hamburg: LIT Verlag.

Taiwo, O. (1993) 'Colonialism and Its Aftermath: The Crisis of Knowledge Production'. Callaloo, 16(4): 891– 908.

Thorpe, S.A. (1993) 'African traditional religions'. Pretoria: University of South Africa.

Ubrurhe, J.O. (2003) 'Urhobo Traditional Medicine'. Ibadan: Spectrum Books Limited.

Westerlund, D. (2006) 'African indigenous religions and disease causation'. Leiden: Brill.

White, P. (2015) 'The concept of diseases and healthcare in African traditional religion in Ghana'. HTS Teologiese Studies/Theological Studies 71(3), Art. #2762. http://dx.doi.org/10.4102/ hts. v71i3.2762.

Chapter 2

Medicine, Culture and Health Belief Systems

The concept and meaning of culture

Culture, as it is usually understood, is the way of life shared by a group of people that claim to share a single origin or descent. It entails a totality of traits and characteristics that are peculiar to a people to the extent that it marks them out from other peoples or societies. These particular traits include the people's language, dress, music, work, arts, religion, dancing and so on, as well as their social norms, taboos and values (Idang, 2015). It embraces the way people walk and how they talk, the manner in which they treat death and greet the new-born. Edward B. Taylor is reputed to be the scholar who first defined culture, in his work "Primitive Culture" (1871, reprinted in 1958). Taylor saw culture as a complex whole which includes knowledge, belief, art, morals, law, customs or any other capabilities and habits acquired by man as a member of society.

Today, there are as many definitions of culture as there are scholars interested in the phenomenon. In an attempt to capture the all-embracing nature of culture, Bello (1991) described it as the totality of the way of life evolved by a people in their attempts to meet the challenge of living in their environment, which gives order and meaning to their social, political, economic, aesthetic and religious norms, thus distinguishing a people from their neighbours. Indeed, the many definitions of culture all have this single underlying characteristic: the attempt to portray culture as the entire or total way of life of a particular group of people. It can also be said that culture is uniquely human and shared with other people in a society.

Culture is selective in what it absorbs or accepts from other people outside a particular cultural group (Idang, 2015). Culture is passed on from generation to generation, and the acquisition of culture is a result of the socialisation process (Fafunwa, 1974). That culture is understood as the way of life of a people presupposes the fact that there can be no people without a culture. To claim that there is a society without a culture would imply that this society has continued to survive without any form of social organisa-tion or institutions, norms, beliefs and taboos – which would be quite untrue. Some Western scholars, who may be tempted to use their own cultural categories to judge distinctively different people as "primitive", may claim that such people have no history, religion or even philosophy, but cannot say that they have no culture.

Culture has been classified into material and non-material aspects. While material culture refers to the visible, tactile objects which are manufactured for the purposes of human survival, non-material culture comprises of the norms and social mores of the people, including taboos and beliefs about what is good and bad. While material culture is concrete and takes the form of artefacts and crafts, non-material culture is abstract but has a very pervasive influence on the lives of the people of a particular culture.

Culture is dynamic; it is continually changing. Antia (2005) states that culture is not fixed and permanent; it is always being changed and modified through contacts with and absorption of other peoples' cultures, in a process known as assimilation. As people change their social patterns and institutions, beliefs and values, and even skills and tools of work, then culture has to be an adaptive system. Each element of a culture is related to the whole system (Etuk, 2002). Once an aspect of culture adjusts or shifts in response to changes from within or outside the environment, then other aspects of the culture are affected, whether directly or indirectly.

Idiong (1994) suggests that there are some widely held misconceptions and negative perceptions about the word culture, causing some people to conjure images of masquerades, idol worshipping, traditional jamborees, magic, voodoo and other activities they consider bizarre. This misconception, we believe, is not widespread but may have arisen from a limited understanding of the meaning of culture. As we shall see, culture generally – and African culture in particular – is like a two-sided coin: it can have negative aspects, but it also has many soul-lifting, life-enhancing and positive dimensions.

This book deals with African culture and draws examples from Nigerian culture. There are of course many cultures in Africa; the continent is inhabited by various ethnic nationalities with different languages, modes of dress, food, dancing and even greeting habits. Obviously, virtually every locality has unique features. Yet notwithstanding the cultural variations that make each local or regional manifestation of culture unique, the cultures value systems and beliefs of traditional African societies are close, and Africans share some dominant traits in their belief systems and have similar values that mark them out from other peoples of the world (Idang, 2015). According to Walter (1973), the continent of Africa south of the great Sahara desert formed a broad community where resemblances were clearly discernible. Certainly African cultures differ vastly from the cultures of other regions or continents, justifying our usage of the term "African culture". A

Nigerian culture, for instance, would be closer to, say, a Ghanaian culture on certain cultural parameters than it would be to the Oriental culture of the Eastern world or to the Western culture of Europe (Idang, 2015).

According to Ezedike (2009), African culture refers to the sum total of shared attitudinal inclinations and capabilities, art, beliefs, moral codes and practices that characterise Africans. It can be conceived of as a continuous, cumulative reservoir containing both material and non-material aspects that are socially transmitted from one generation to another.

African traditional beliefs on health and causes of disease

Traditional African belief systems are characterised by strong faith in spiritual powers. The word "spiritual", as seen in aspects of the biopsychosocial approach(es) to healthcare and illness (Mbiti, 1970; Kiev, 1964), is based on beliefs which can be connected to the history and culture of Africa (Mbiti, 1970). The behaviour of Africans is motivated by what they believe, and what they believe is based on what they experience. Although Western medicine and health care systems have been introduced in Africa, many African countries still rely on traditional health care (Osei, 2004; Iroegbu, 2005; Lambo, 1964).

By way of free will, humans make choices based on many factors, including their spiritual beliefs, preferences, knowledge and perceptions (Anthony, 2003). In Africa, spiritual belief is a major determinant of choice of treatment (Osei, 2004). A belief system based on Creationism (i.e. the religious belief that the Almighty God created the universe and the first man, rather than the scientific conclusion that they were created by natural processes) is strongly held by indigenous Africans (Mbiti, 1970, Danquah, 2014). The continued widespread existence of spiritual belief among Africans suggests its heritability, but in fact it is transferred from one generation to another. There are different kinds of beliefs – the belief in the Almighty God and belief in other spirits (Mbiti, 1970; Appiah et al., 2007; Omonzejele, 2008; Kiev, 1964). As this continues to run across generations, spiritual belief in Africa can be described as a form of 'behaviour genetics'.

In Africa, many herbalists prepare their herbs on the basis of spiritual belief. The elite African who has knowledge about the scientific cause of illness also incorporates spiritual factors when dealing with illnesses. The current Western model, the biopsychosocial model considers health as including physical, mental, emotional and social factors (Engel, 1980). For the African, however, wellbeing is not just about the healthy functioning of the body system through proper healthcare and lifestyle, but goes beyond scientific causes to include spiritual involvement (Mbiti, 1970; Kiev, 1964).

The modification of the biopsychosocial model to include spiritual factors (McKee and Chappel, 1992) is therefore well suited to the African culture.

For the traditional African, good health consists of mental, physical, spiritual and emotional stability not only of oneself, but also of one's family members and community. This integrated view of health is based on the African unitary view of reality (Omonzejele, 2008). Good health is also often understood in terms of the relationship with one's ancestors. For many Africans, it is of paramount importance that ancestors stay healthy so that they can protect the living (Iroegbu, 2005). Good health is also believed to be a result of appropriate behaviour—that is, living in accordance with the values and norms of the society (Iroegbu, 2005). In view of the above, traditional medicine has at its base a deep-rooted belief in the interaction between people's spiritual and physical wellbeing (Setswe, 1999). It is imperative to emphasise the significance for health of this perception of the individual as a member of the collective community; as such, good health is dependent on good relations with community. Mbiti (1990: pp 108-109) notes that:

> *Only in terms of the other people does the individual become conscious of his own being ... When he suffers, he does not suffer alone but with the corporate group ... Whatever happens to the individual happens to the whole group, and whatever happens to the whole group happens to the individual. The individual can only say: I am because we are, and since we are, therefore I am.*

Traditional African beliefs include several ways to explain or understand the causes of disease. The first is the view that disease is often caused by attacks from evil or bad spirits. Some also believe that if the ancestors are not treated well, they may punish people with disease (Magesa, 1997; Westerlund, 2006). African traditional religion is thus based on maintaining the balance between the visible and invisible world. The maintenance of this balance and, 1997; Westerlund, 2006). African traditional religion is thus based on maintaining the balance between the visible and invisible world. The maintaining of this balance and harmony is humanity's greatest ethical obligation, and determines quality of life (Magesa, 1997). Nyamiti (1984: p.16) pointed out:

> *When ancestors are neglected or forgotten by their relatives they are said to be angry with them and to send them misfortunes as punishment. Their anger is usually appeased through prayers and ritual in the form of food and drinks.*

Good behaviour, according to African traditional belief, includes respecting and practising the values established by society and culture, participating in religious rituals and practices, and showing proper respect for family, neighbours and the community. Failure to follow these behavioural guidelines often results in good spirits withdrawing their blessing and protection, thereby opening doors to illness, death, drought or other misfortune.

Spell-casting and witchcraft are other reasons used to explain ill-health. There is a view that people with evil powers can punish their enemies or those who are disrespectful to them by causing them to become sick (Olupona, 2004). Furthermore, many traditional African communities believe that certain illnesses which defy scientific treatment can be transmitted through witchcraft and unforeseen forces; these include infertility, attacks by dangerous animal, snake bites, persistent headaches and repeated miscarriages (Obinna, 2012, Thorpe, 1993). In some Ghanaian communities, especially in Akan communities, it is believed that a person can become sick as a result of the invocation of curses in the name of the river deity, Antoa, which is seen as a means of seeking divine justice (White, 2015).

Many traditional healers and practitioners believe that sickness results from disregarding taboos (Gyekye, 1995), Taboos form an important part of African traditional religion. They are behaviours, practices or lifestyles that are forbiden by a community or a group of people (Isiramen, 1998). Taboos encompass social or religious customs prohibiting or restricting a particular practice, or forbidding association with a particular person, place or thing (Westerlund, 2006). Magesa (1997) asserted that taboos exist to ensure that the moral structures of the universe remain undisturbed for the good of humanity. It is believed that when a person violates any taboo, whether openly or in secret, the consequences always manifest either in the person(s) concerned, or in the entire community, in the form of diseases, and possibly death. This is what Magesa (1997) termed the "effect of life force", arguing that moral behaviour maintains and enhances one's life force, but disobedience and disloyal behaviour towards traditions passed on by the ancestors will weaken the life force, leading to punishment from the ancestors or spirits in the form of disease and misfortune.

According to Wiredu (1980), among the Akan people of Ghana, morality is based on human welfare, while Downess (1977) indicates that the African idea of morality is based on doing good to others and not evil. African notions and application of moral precepts have far-reaching implications for how African traditional medicine is practiced. Adherence to moral precepts is an important and integral part of traditional health care in Africa and is subsumed in African ethics.

Patients' individual health beliefs can have a profound impact on their clinical care, as explored further below. They can impede preventive efforts, delay or complicate medical care, and result in the use of folk remedies that can be beneficial or toxic. Culturally based attitudes to seeking treatment and trusting traditional medicines and folk remedies are rooted in core belief systems regarding illness causation, e.g. naturalistic Ayurvedic and biomedical. Read (1966) observed that in African systems, there are three groups of illness: trivial or everyday complaints treated by home remedies; "European disease" – that is, disease that responds to Western scientific therapy; and "African disease" – disease that is not likely to be understood or treated successfully by Western medicine. This observation, according to Oke and Owumi (1996), is true for many ethnic groups in Nigeria. Erinosho (1976) and Oke (1995), working among Yorubas and Owumi (1989) among the Okpe people of Delta State, noted that illness etiology could be traced to three basic factors: natural, supernatural and mystical.

Illness is not only a personal affair; it also arouses a wide variety of feelings in those close to the sufferer as they engage in a search for treatment, which becomes an immediate problem (Onu, 1999). According to Onu, for the patient a serious illness carries with it the underlying fear of death or permanent disability, and constitutes a crisis which requires cooperative efforts both from family members and health care providers (physical or spiritual).

Influence of cultural beliefs on health and illness behaviour

All cultures have systems of health beliefs to explain what causes illness, how it can be cured or treated, and who should be involved in the process (McLaughlin and Braun, 1998). Research has extended the description of illness beyond actual diseases to include how the sick person, and the members of the family or wider social network perceive, live with, and respond to symptoms and disability (Kleinman, 1988). Kleinman argued that the illness experience includes categorising and explaining the forms of distress caused by those physiological processes. It therefore follows that any productive effort to improve the wellbeing of patients must include an understanding of their perception of illness and its symptoms.

When patients are diagnosed with an illness, they generally develop an organised pattern of beliefs about their condition. These views are key determinants of behaviour directed at managing illness, and change in response to shifts in patients' perceptions and ideas about their illness. These illness perceptions or cognitive representations directly influence the individual's emotional response to the illness as well as their coping behaviour, such as adherence to treatment. Yet despite their importance, patients' views about their illness or symptoms are rarely sought in medical interviews, and patients tend not to discuss their illness beliefs with doctors. Understanding common perceptions in indigenous communities about the causes of ill-health may help policy-makers to design effective integrated primary healthcare strategies to serve these communities (Mesfin et al., 2017).

Illness is commonly described as a condition of pronounced deviation from the normal healthy state. The term is often used to mean disease, but can also refer to a person's perception of their health, regardless of whether they have a disease or not. A person without any disease may feel unhealthy and simply have the perception of having a disease, while another person would experience the same condition as feeling healthy (Vaughnet al., 2009). Johnson, (2002) argued that illnesses cannot be investigated solely by the methods of biomedicine because its study ultimately depends directly on phenomenological analysis of experienced suffering through individual self-reports and behaviour, and therefore its presence cannot be objectively established by physical signs.

According to Petrie and Weinman (2012), patients' models of their illness share a common structure; this is made up of beliefs about the cause of the illness, the symptoms that are part of the condition, the consequences for the patient's life, how the illness is controlled or cured, and how long the illness will last. These beliefs are based either on a patient's own medical knowledge and experience, or on the experiences of friends or family members who have had similar symptoms or diagnoses (Broadbent et al., 2006). Patients with the same illness may have different perceptions of their condition and different emotional reactions to it. Interventions based around changing, inaccurate or unhelpful perceptions of illness are an important emerging area of health psychology. It is important to note that patients' knowledge of medical concepts and the body is often rudimentary, limiting the accuracy and complexity of the models they build. Nevertheless, as stated above, a patient's perception of their illness can influence their coping ability, compliance with treatment and functional recovery. Psychological interventions to address negative beliefs and perceptions may facilitate an earlier return to work (Giriet al., 2009).

People routinely experience symptoms that may signal illness, such as lethargy, depression, anorexia, sleepiness, hyperalgesia, and inability to concentrate. While symptoms are critical elements in a person's decision to seek medical attention, the presence of symptoms is not always sufficient to prompt a visit to doctor . Some people seek help for symptoms, while others do not. When people seek and perceive symptoms of illness, they often consult others such as friends, neighbours or family members on whether or not to report the symptoms to a doctor. Some may be advised not do so until their condition worsens. Some deny the symptoms, while others resort to self-medication. Some go to "quacks" (bogus doctors) and may not be properly treated. Mechanic (1968) listed characteristics that determine perceptions of symptoms, as follows: (i) The visibility of the symptoms, that is, how readily apparent they are; (ii) Perceived severity of the symptoms. Symptom perceived as severe will be more likely to prompt action than less severe ones; (iii) The extent to which symptoms interfere with personal life. A greater extent will prompt an individual to seek medical care as quickly as possible; and (iv) The frequency and persistency of the symptoms. Conditions that people view as requiring care tend to be those that are severe and continuous; intermittent symptoms are less likely to generate illness behaviour. According to Robert and Pennebaker (1995), severe symptoms prompt people to seek help from friends, family and physicians, though even mild symptoms prompt people to seek help when they persist.

Certain biomedical etiologies maintain that symptoms are the manifestation of bodily malfunction, whereas in non-orthodox health care systems, symptoms are believed to be manifestations of the intrusion of the supernatural (Chipfakacha, 1994). Most cultures support the belief that symptoms are the manifestation of illness, whether it is caused by a pathogen or a spirit invasion. Therefore, in order to effectively treat these illnesses, remedies must be both material (e.g. herbal remedy) and spiritual (e.g. amulets) (Vaughn et al., 2009). Further, social support has been found to have significant influence on subjective wellbeing (Kahn et al., 2003). Other research findings also hold that social support seems to exert an influence on health, both directly and indirectly, through certain cognitive mechanisms, coping strategies and health behaviours (Cohen and Wills, 1985).

It can be concluded that, whatever a patient's cultural belief may be, how the patient perceives his/her illness will affect the patient's rate of recovery and response to treatment. It is therefore recommended that health practitioners focus attention on patients' perceptions of their illness symptoms, and provide social and psychological support in order to aid the patient's recovery and improve their response to treatment.

References

Adjaye, J.K. (2001) 'The performativity of Akan libations: An ethnopoetic construction of reality'. Ghana Studies 4, 107–138.

Anthony, D.J. (2003) 'Psychotherapies in counselling'. Bangalore, India: Anugraha Publications.

Antia, O.R.U. (2005) 'Akwa Ibom Cultural Heritage: Its Incursion by Western Culture and its Renaissance'. Uyo: Abbny Publishers.

Appiah P., Appiah K.A. and Agyeman-Duah I. (2007) 'Proverbs of the Akans: Bu Me Bɛ'. Oxfordshire: Ayebia Clarke Publishing Ltd, p. 336.

Aziza, R.C. (2001) 'The Relationship between Language use and Survival of Culture: the case of Umobo youth'. Nigerian Language Studies. No. 4.

Bello, S. (1991) 'Culture and Decision Making in Nigeria'. Lagos: National Council for Arts and Culture.

Berg, A. (2003) 'Ancestor reverence and mental health in South Africa'. Transcultural Psychiatry. 2003; 40(2): 194–207. [PubMed: 12940645] Boeree, C.G. [4 April 2008] Personality theories. n.d. Available at: http:// www.ship.edu/~cgboeree/ kelly.html.

Broadbent, E., Petrie K.J., Main, J. and Weinmann, J. (2006) 'The brief illness perception questionnaire'. Journal of Psychosomatic Research, 60, 631– 637.

Brooks, G.E. (2003) 'Eurafricansinwestern Africa: commerce, socialstatus, gender, and religious observance from the sixteenth to the eighteenth century'. Western African studies. Athens, OH: Ohio University Press.

Chavunduka, G.L.(1999) 'Christianity, African religion and African medicine'. World Courncil of Churches, viewed 23 August 2017, at http:// wcc-coe.org/wcc/what/ interreligious/cd33-02.html

Chipfakacha V. (1994) 'The role of culture in primary health care'. South African Medical Journal 84(12): 860–1.

Chuke, P.O. (1988) 'Nigeria'. In: R.B. Saltman (ed.) The International Handbook of Health Care Systems. N.Y: Greenwood Press.

Cohen, S. and Wills, T.A. (1985) 'Stress, Social Support and the Buffering Hypothesis'. Psychological Bulletin, 98, 310–357.

Craffert, P.F. 'Opposing world-views: The border guards between traditional and biomedical health care practices'. South African Journal of Ethnology. 1997; 20(1):1–8.

Danquah, S.A. (2014) 'Clinical psychology in Ghana: history, training, research and practice'. Saarbrucken: Lambert Academic Publishing.

Davidson, B. (1998) 'West Africa before the colonial era: a history to 1850'. London: Longman.

Downess, R.M. (1977) 'TIV religion', Ibadan: University of Ibadan Press. Engel, G.L. (1980) 'The clinical application of the biopsychosocial model'. AMJ Psychiatry 137: 535–544.

Etuk, U.A. (2002) 'Religion and Cultural Identity'. Ibadan: Hope Publication.

Ezedike, E.O. (2009) 'African Culture and the African Personality. From Footmarks to Landmarks on African Philosophy'. Somolu: Obaroh and Ogbinaka Publishers.

Fafunwa, A.B. (1974) 'History of Education in Nigeria'. London: George Allen and Unwin.

Giri, P., Poole J., Nightingale P. and Robertson, A. (2009). 'Perceptions of illness and their impact on illness absence'. Occup Med (Lond) (2009) 59 (8): 550-555. doi:10.1093/occmed/kqp123

Gyekye, K. (1995) 'African philosophical thought: The Akan conceptual scheme', rev. edn., Philadelphia, PA:Temple University Press.

Haines, W.D. (2005) 'Cultural Anthropology: Adaptations, Structures and Meanings'. Upper Saddle River, NJ: Pearson – Prentice Hall.

Idang, G.E. (2015) Phronimon Volume 16 | Number 2 | 2015 pp. 97–111. ISSN 1561-4018 © Unisa Press.

Idiong, S.O. (1994) 'Culture in Education'. In Sociology of Education: A Book of Readings. Calabar: Edigraph Communications.

Idowu, B. (1973) 'African traditional religion: A definition' London:SCM. Iroegbu, E.P. (2005a) 'Iga n'ajuju: Igbo Ways of Questioning'. In: Gottschalk-Batschkus, C.E. and Green, J.C. (eds.) Ethnotherapies in Cycle of Life – Fading, Being and Becoming. Munchen-Germany: Institute for Ethnomedicine.

Iroegbu, E.P. (2005b) 'Healing insanity: Skills and expert knowledge of Igbo healers', African Development 30(3), 78–92. http://dx.doi.org/10.4314/ad.v30i3.22231.

Isiramen, C. (1998) 'Philosophy of religion, ethics and early church controversies'.Lago: AB Associate Publishers.

Johnson, R. (2002) 'The concept of illness behavior: a brief chronological account of four key discoveries'. Veterinary Immunology and Immunopathology, 87 (3–4): 443450.doi:10.1016/ S0165-2427(02)00069–7.

Kahissay, M.H., Fenta, T.G. and Boon, H. 'Beliefs and perception of ill-health causation: a socio-cultural qualitative study in rural North-Eastern Ethiopia'. BMC Public Health.2017 Jan 26. doi: 10.1186/ s12889-017- 4052-y.

Kahn, J.H., Hessling, R.M. and Russell, D.W. (2003) 'Social support, health, and well being among the elderly: What is the role of negative affectivity?' Personality and Individual Differences 35, 5–17.

Kiev A. (1964) 'Magic, faith and health'. NY, USA: The Free Press.

Kleinman, A. (1988) 'The illness narratives: suffering, healing, and the human condition'. New York: Basic Books.

Lambo T.A. (1964) 'Patterns of psychiatric care in developing African countries'. (Ari Kiev Edn) Magic, faith and health. NY, USA: The Free Press.

Magesa, L. (1997) 'African religion: The moral traditions of abundant life'. Maryknoll, NY: Orbis Books

Mbiti J.S. (1970) 'Concepts of God in Africa'. London: The Camelot Press Ltd, p. 348.

Mbiti, J.S. (1990) 'African religions and philosophy', London: Heinemann. McLaughlin, L. and Braun, K. (1998) 'Asian and Pacific Islander cultural values: Considerations for health care decision-making'. Health and Social Work, 23(2), 116–126.

McKee D.D. and Chappel J.N. (1992) 'Spirituality and medical practice'. J Fam Pract 35: 205–208.

Mechanic, D. (1968) 'Medical Sociology'. New York: Free Press.

Metz H.C. (ed.) 'Nigeria: A Country Study'. Washington: GPO for the Library of Congress, 1991.

Nyamiti, C. (1984) 'Christ as our ancestor: Christology from an African perspective'. Gweru: Mambo Press.

Obinna, E. (2012) 'Life is a superior to wealth?: Indigenous healers in an African community, Amariri, Nigeria', in A. Afe, E. Chitando & B.

Bateye (eds.) African traditions in the study of religion in Africa. Farnham: Ashgate Publishing, pp. 137–139.

Oke, E.A. (1995) 'Traditional Health Services: An Investigation of Providers and the Level and Pattern of Utilization among the Yoruba'. Ibadan Sociological Series, No. 1: 2–5.

Oke, E.A. and Owumi, B.E. (1996) Readings in Medical Sociology. Ibadan: Adjacent Press.

Olupona, J.K. (2004) 'Owner of the day and regulator of the universe: Ifa Divination and healing among the Yoruba of South-Western Nigeria' in M. Winkelman and P.M. Peeks (eds.) Divination and healing: Potent vision, pp.103–117. Tucson, AZ: University of Arizona Press.

Omonzejele, P.F. (2008) 'African concepts of health, disease, and treatment: An ethical inquiry', Explore 4(2), 120–123. http://dx.doi. org/10.1016/j. explore.2007.12.001.

Onu, A.O. (1999) 'Social Basis of Illness: A Search for Therapeutic Meaning' in Okpoko, A.I. (ed). Africa's Indigenous Technology. Ibadan: Wisdom Publishers Ltd.

Osei, A.O. (2004) 'Types of psychiatric illnesses at traditional healing centres in Ghana'. Gh Med J 35: 106–110.

Parfitt, R.T. (1978) 'Drug Discovery, Design or Serendipity. An Inaugural Lecture Series'. University of Bath, UK.

Petrie, K.J. and Weinmann, J. (2006) 'Why illness perceptions matter'. Clinical Medicine, 6, 536–539.

Petrie, K.J. and Weinman, J. (2012). 'Patients' Perceptions of Their Illness: The Dynamo of Volition in Health Care'. Current Directions in Psychological Science, 21(1), 60–65

Read, M. (1966) 'Culture, Health and Disease, Social and Cultural Influences on Health Programmes in Developing Countries'. USA: Tavistock Publishers.

Rodney, W. (1972) 'How Europe Underdeveloped Africa'. London: Bogle-L'Ouverture Publications.

Setswe, G. (1999) 'The role of traditional healers and primary health care in South Africa'. Health SA Gesondheid 4(2), 56–60. http://dx.doi. org/10.4102/hsag. v4i2.356.

Smith, T. (1998) 'Complete Family Health Encyclopedia'. London: Dorling Kindersley.

Taylor, E.B. (1871) 'Primitive Culture: Researches into the Development of Mythology, Philosophy, Religion, Language, Art and Custom'. 2nd ed. London: John Murray.

Teuton, J., Bentall, R. and Dowrick, C. (2007) 'Conceptualizing psychosis in Uganda: The perspective of indigenous and religious healers'. Transcultural Psychiatry. 2007; 44(1):79–114. [PubMed: 17379612].

Thorpe, S.A. (1993) 'African traditional religions'. Pretoria: University of South Africa.

Vaughn, L.M., Jacquez, F. and Baker, R.C. (2009) 'Cultural Health Attributions, Beliefs, and Practices: Effects on Healthcare and Medical Education'. The Open Medical Education Journal, 2009, 2, 64–74.

Westerlund, D. (2006) 'African indigenous religions and disease causation'. Leiden: Brill.

White, P. (2015) 'The concept of diseases and health care in African traditional religion in Ghana'. HTS Teologiese Studies/Theological Studies 71(3), Art. #2762. http://dx.doi.org/10.4102/ hts. v71i3.2762.

Wiredu, K. (1980) 'Philosophy and an African Culture'. London: Cambridge University Press.

WHO (1978) Alma-Ata Primary Health Care. Geneva: World Health Organization.

Chapter 3

Trees

Trees refer to woody perennial plants, typically having a single stem or trunk growing to a considerable height and bearing lateral branches at some distance from the ground. Many of these trees are used by local communities in Nigeria and Africa for various medicinal purposes. This chapter examines how these trees are traditionally used for medicinal purposes and also attempts to show the scientific basis of their uses.

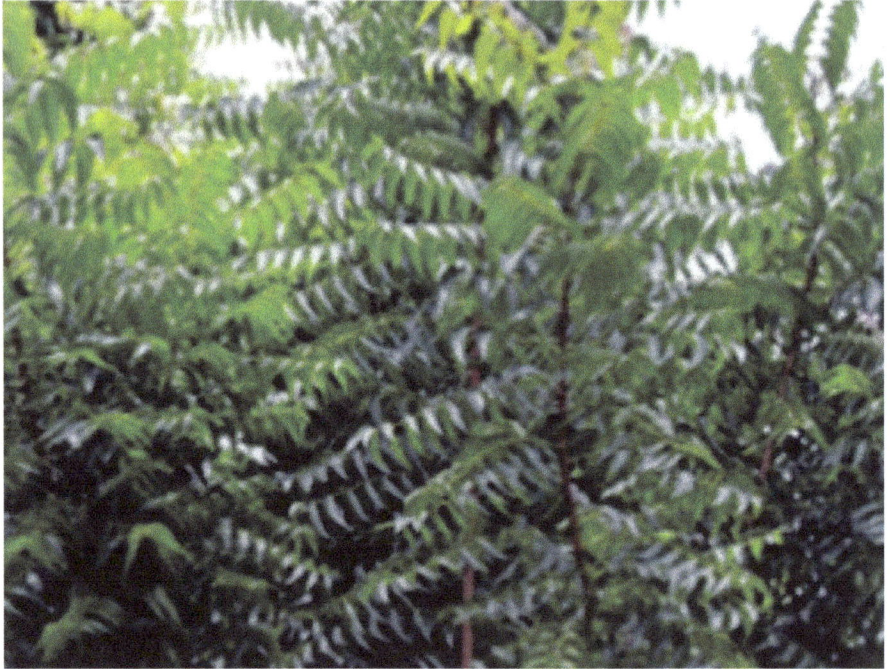

Family: Meliaceae

Botanical Name: *Azadirachta Indica*

Common Names: NeemTree (dongoyaro)

Local Name: *Edo:* Ebe-dongoyaro *Igbo:* Ogwu akom *Hausa:* Dongoyaro *Yoruba:* Aforo-oyinbo

History: Neem tree is mainly cultivated in the Indian subcontinent.

Belief: Neem products are believed by Siddha andAyurvedic practitioners to be anthelmintic, antifungal, antidiabetic, antibacterial, antiviral, contraceptive.

Parts Used: Leaves, Seeds, Roots and Bark

Local Uses: The leaves and stem bark are used in treating malaria. Particularly prescribed for skin diseases (Zillur Rahman *et al.,* 1996). Vein is used for treating measles and chicken pox (Zillur Rahman *et al.,* 1996). Neem oil is also used for Maverlaria and to balance blood sugar levels (Chopra *et al.,* 1956).

Chemical Constituents: Nimbin, nimbinin, nimbidin, azadirachtin (Heuzé, 2015).

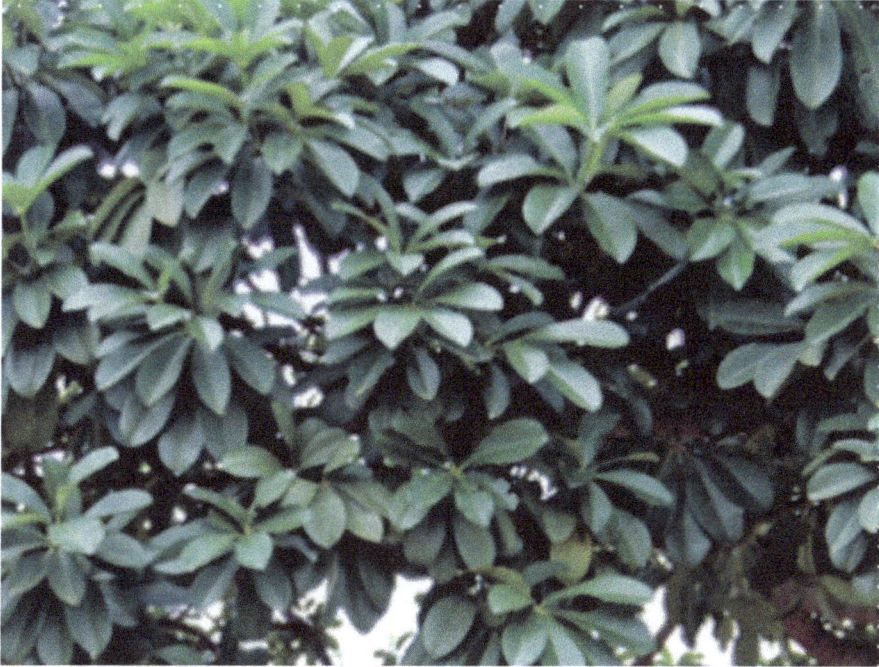

Family: Apocynaceae

Botanical Name: *Alstonia boonei*

Common Names: Stool Wood, Pattern Wood

Local names: *Edo:* Ukhu *Igbo;* Egbe, egbwu-ora. *Yoruba:* Ahun. **Efik**: Ndodo. **Ijaw**: Egbu. **Kwale**: Egbu

History: It is native to tropical West Africa,with arrange extending to Ethiopia and Tanzania.

Belief: Africans regards it as a sacred tree and it is worshipped in the forest hence the parts are not cut off.

Parts Used: Leaves, Latex, Bark, Root

Local Uses: The bark and leaves are used for malaria, asthma and pains. The latex is also used as anasthesia for pain relieve. It is used for treating arthritis (Kweio-Okai,1991)

Chemical Constituents: Alkaloids, Saponin, Tannins, Echitamine, Echtamidine (Burkhill, 1985; Arulmozhi, 2010; Maiza-Benabdesselam et al., 2007).

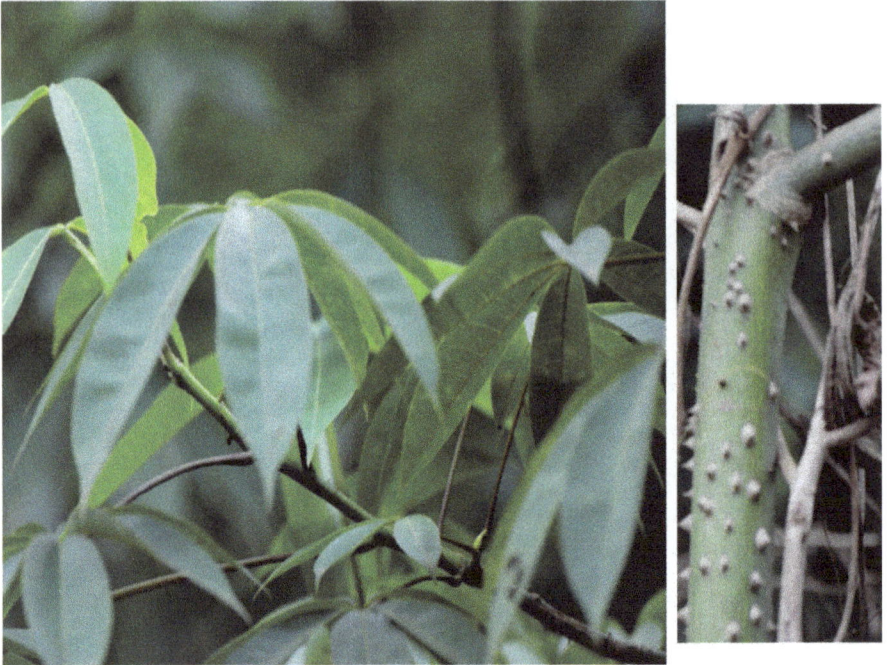

Family: Malvaceae

Botanical name: *Bombax boenopozens*

Common names: West African bombax, Bombax, Ceiba, red silk cotton, red flowered silk cotton tree, Goid coast bombax

Local name: *Edo:* Obokha, Ogi-ugbogha, Olikharo, Ugbogha, *Hausa:* Gujfiyaa, kuryaa, *Igbo:* Akpu, Ngara akpu, Akpu-obololo, Atunjaka. *Yoruba:* Eso, Ponpola, Olokododo

History: It is native to western Africa, the Indian subcontinent, Southeast Asia, as well as subtropical regions of East Asia and northern Australia. It is distinguished from the genus Ceiba which has white flowers.

Beliefs: In many parts of West Africa forest and areas and specific trees are protected and valued for particular cultural occasions and as historic symbols. Each community has its own traditions associated with sacred areas and, as a result, the species that are found in them vary greatly. In analysis of traditional African political institutions, Niangoran-Bouah (1983) notes that there are two traditional sacred locations for reunion: sacred groves and "arbresapalabre." The "arbresapalabre" is the venue for political and social meetings: the location where elders sit under the big tree and talk until they agree.

It is the location where political, judicial, and social decisions are made. Visse (1975) notes that in Côted'Ivoire there are specific tree species which serve as"arbresapalabre" such as *Microdesmis sp.* Blighia sapida (also a symbol of fecundity), Cordia millenii, and *Bombaxbuonopozens.* The bark is burnt to produce a smoke that is believed to drive away evil spirits called *aliziniin* Dagbani.

Local Uses: Both the flowers and the young fruits are used in making soup.

Chemical Constituents: Alkaloids, flavonoids, tannins, saponins, terpenoids, steroids, phlobatannins, anthraquinones and carbohydrates found mostly in the roots (Firempong *et al.,* 2016).

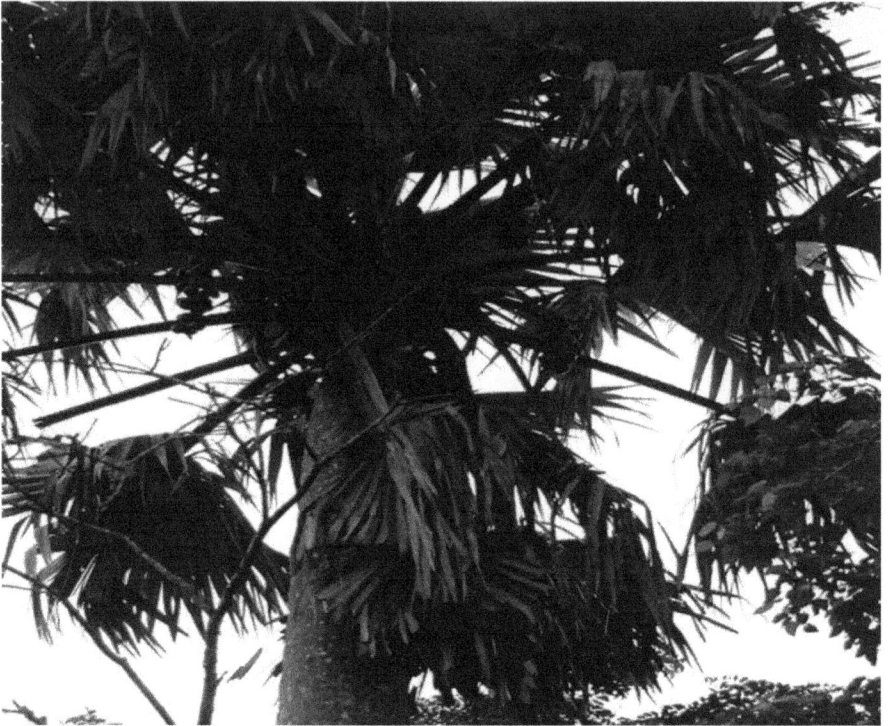

Family: Arecaceae

Botanical name: *Borasus aethiopicum*

Common name: African fan palm, African palmyra palm, deleb palm, ron palm, toddy palm, black rhun palm, ronier palm.

History: *Borassus aethiopum* is a species of Borassus palm from Africa. It is widespread across much of tropical Africa from Senegal to Ethiopia and south to northern South Africa, though it is largely absent from the forested areas of Central Africa and desert regions such as the Sahara and Namib. This palm also grows in northwest Madagascar and the comoros.

Belief: They are believed to play a significant role in rituals and oracles as sacred objects in Africa.

Local uses: The tree has many uses: the fruits are edible, as are the tender roots produced by the young plant; fibres can be osbtained from the leaves; and the wood (which is reputed to be termite-proof) it is also used in construction (Reynolds, 1921: Bailey and Bailey, 1976). The leaves and roots are antidiabetic (Pradeep *et al.,* 2015).

Chemical constituents: Tannins, anthocyanes, saponosides, mucilages, coumarins (Aguzue *et al.,* 2012)

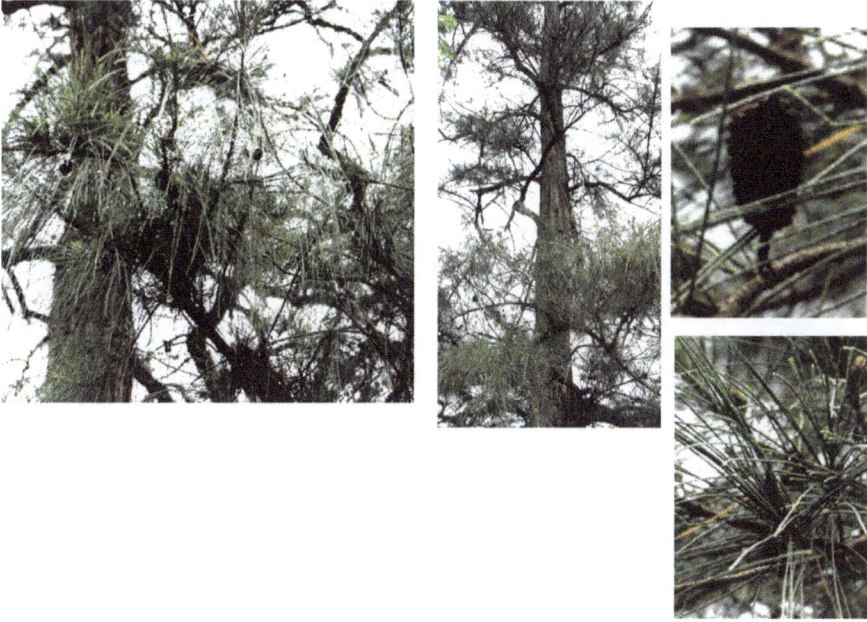

Family: Casuarinaceae

Botanical name: *Casuarina equisetifolia*

Common name: Australian pine tree and Sheoak.

History: The plant is native to Burma, Vietnam, Malaysia, New Caledonia, Vanuatu and Australia. It is also found in Madagascar, but it is doubtful if this is within the native range of the species (Boland *et al.*, 2006).

Belief: The legendary miraculous spear Kaumaile came with the hero Tefolaha on the South Pacific island Nanumea. He fought with it on the islands of Samoa and Tonga. As Tefolaha died, "Kaumaile" went to his heirs, then to their heirs, and on and on for 23 generations. It is about 1.80 meters long and about 880 years old and the tree was cut on Samoa (Sdsee-Speer, 2014).

Local uses: Extracts of leaves exhibit anticancer properties. Bark is astringent and used for stomach ache, diarrhoea, dysentery and nervous disorders. The Seeds are anthelmintic, antispasmodic and antidiabetic (Ahsan et al., 2009; Jain and Dam, 1979).

Chemical constituents: Alkaloids, steroids, carbohydrates, tannins, fixed oils, proteins, triterpenoids, deoxysugar, flavonoid, cyanogenetic and coumarin glycosides (Khandelwal and Nirali, 2006).

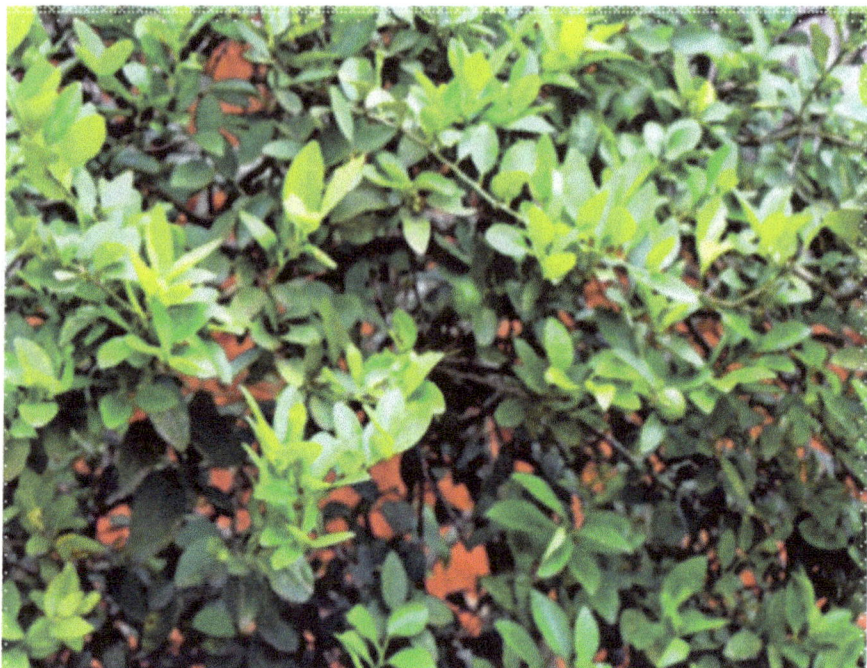

Family: Rutaceae

Botanical name: *Citrus aurantifolia*

Common names: Lime, Bitter orange, Seville orange, sour orange, bigarade orange, or marmalade orange.

Local names: *Yoruba:* Osan ghanhinghanhin, *Igbo:* Olomaoyinbo, *Hausa:* Babban lemu

History: The name comes from its association with Florida keys, where it is best known as the flavouring ingredients in key lime pie.

Parts used: leaves, fruits, peel and oil.

Local uses: The leaves are used as tea for bilious head ache. Fresh juice is also used to counter diarrhoea. It is used to lighten the skin. It stimulates the digestive system, detoxifies the body, cools fever and is used in treating rheumatic pain. It has an a strigent action, clears congested skin and stops bleeding from minor cuts. (Aibinu et al., 2006; Nwankwo *et al.,* 2015; Pathan *et al.,* 2012).

Chemical constituents: essential oils, apigenin, hesperetin, kaempferol, nobiletin, quercetin, and rutin (Kawaii *et al.,* 1999; Caristi *et al.,* 2003).

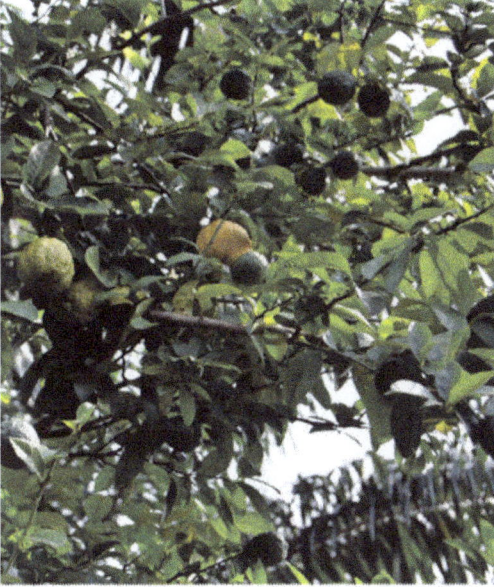

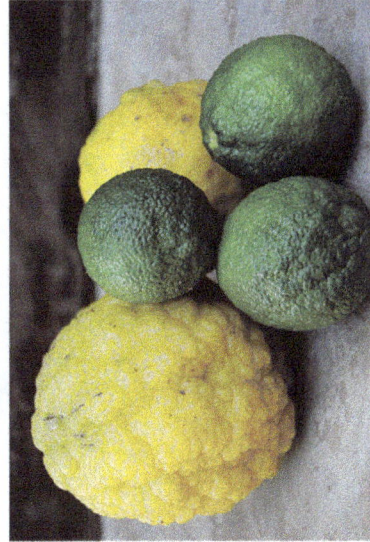

Family: Rutaceae

Botanical name: *Citrus limon*

Common names: Lemon

Local name: *Yoruba:* Osan wewe, *Igbo:* Olomankilisi, *Hausa:* Lemunoisami

History: *Citrus limon,* lemon, is a small tree in the Rutaceae (citrus family) that originated in Asia (likely India and Pakistan)

Belief: There is a belief in Ayurvedic medicine that a cup of hot water with lemon juice in it detoxifies and purifies the liver.

Parts used: Leaves and fruits.

Local uses: Lemon juice helps to control blood pressure, purifies the blood, reduces swollen spleen and strengthens the immune system as it has vitamins C, B2, calcium, iron etc. It protects body against germs and bacteria. It is used for bronchitis, ear ache, nose bleeding, hepatitis, gastric ulcer, menorrhagia. It helps prevents scurvy, whooping cough, cold etc. Lemon oil may be used in aromatherapy (Kiecolt-Glaser *et al.,* 2008; Cooke and Ernst, 2000).

Chemical constituents: Flavonoid, limonoid and citric acid (Penniston *et al.,* 2008; Rauf *et al.*, 2014).

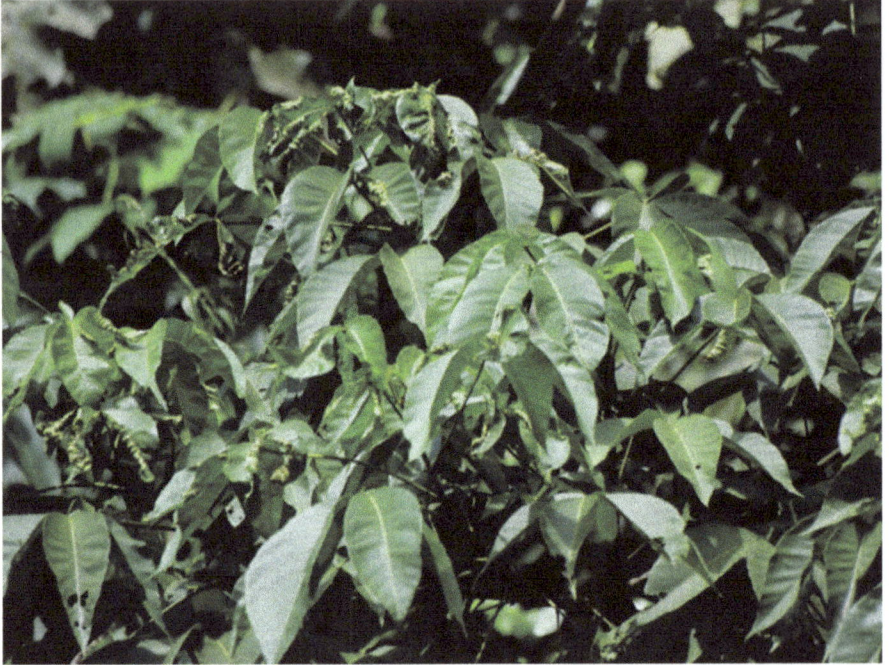

Family: Araliaceae

Botanical name: *Cussiona barteri*

Common name: Octopus cabbage tree

Local Name: *Benin:* Evbi-nato. ***Fulani:*** Takandargiwa. ***Hausa:*** Bumarlahi. ***Yoruba:*** Sigosiga; Sigosego

History: It is commonly found in Africa (Beentje, 1994).

Belief: Because of the likeness of the defoliated tree to deformed limbs, and based on the 'Doctrine of Signatures', the plant is often used in Africa in the treatment of leprosy. Most commonly, the stem is macerated and taken as a purgative and is also applied externally as a lotion; the leprous sores may also be dressed with the powdered stem-bark. The leafy twigs are used with magical rites in the treatment of yellow fever, oedemas, paralysis and sleeping-sickness.

Local Uses: The water in which the leaves have been boiled is purgative and is taken as a remedy for constipation. The pulped up young shoots are eaten as a remedy for diarrhoea.

A decoction of the leaves is used as an eye-wash for treating conjunctivitis, and as a massage in cases of epilepsy in both adults and children. The plant is an emeto-purgative and diuretic, and these cleansing actions upon the body are used in the treatment of various complaints. The plant is also prescribed as a poison-antidote and is used in the treatment of fevers (De Villiers *et al.,* 2010).

Chemical constituents: Cussonosides A and B, two triterpene-saponins, phenol, flavonoid and tanin (Cowan, 1999; Agbor et al., 2004).

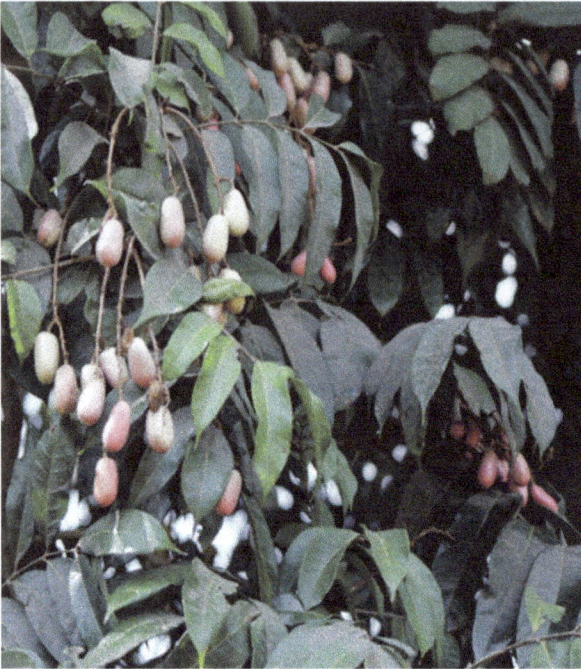

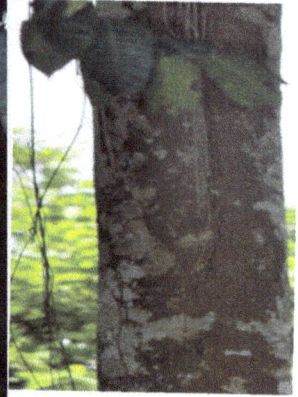

Family: Burseraceae

Botanical name: *Dacryodesedulis*

Common name: Native pear, African plum, blush butter tree, African-pear.

Local name: *Edo:* Orunmwunn *Igbo:* Ube-igbo, ube, Ube-umbu, ubenkputaki, *Yoruba:* Elemi

History: It is a tree native to West Africa, sometimes called Atangain Gabon (National Research Council, 2008).

Belief: Africans believed that Leopard meat can only be eaten if it is exorcised under a safou tree in a public place. This tradition is based on the belief that leopards, like other mammals which kill and eat humans are cursed. The fruit of the tree under which the exorcism is carried out are forbidden to women.

Local uses: It has long been used in the traditional medicine of some African countries to treat various ailments such as wound, skin diseases, dysentery and fever (Omonhinmin *et al.,* 2013).

Chemical Constituents: Terpenes, flavonoids, tannins, alkaloids and saponins palmitic acids, oleic acids and Linoleic acids (Ajibesin, 2011)

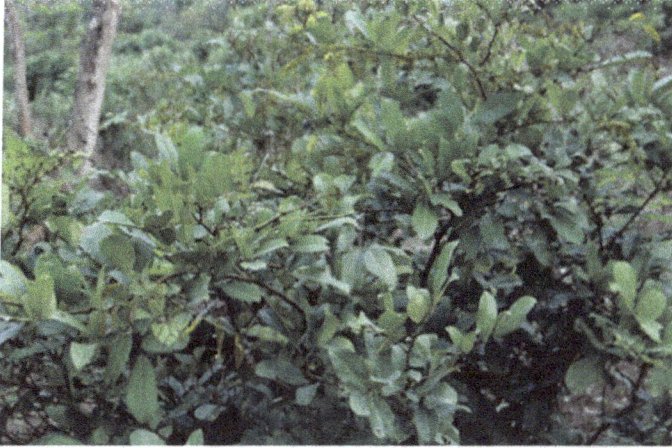

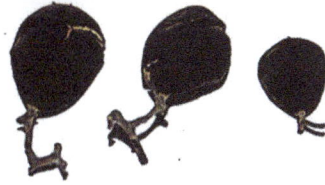

Family: Fabaceae

Botanical name: *Dialum guineense*

Common names: Velvet or black tamarind

Local names: *Yoruba:* Awin, *Igbo*: Icheku, *Hausa:* Tsamiyar Kurm

History: It grows in dense forests in Africa along the southern edge of the Sahel. In Togo.it is called atchethewh. The velvet tamarind can be found in West African countries such as Ghana, Sierra Leone, Senegal, Guinea-Bissau and Nigeria.

Parts used: whole plant

Local uses: It is used for diarrhoea. Infusion of the leaves and fruits it used to treat fever. Twigs are chewed for cleaning teeth. Decoction and infusion of the bark is used for stomach ache, tooth ache, as a gargle and mouth wash. Root are considered aphrodisiac (Burkill, 1985).

Chemical constituents: Tannins, steroids, terpenes, alkaloids flavonoids, saponin, and phenolic compounds (Utubaku *et al.,* 2017).

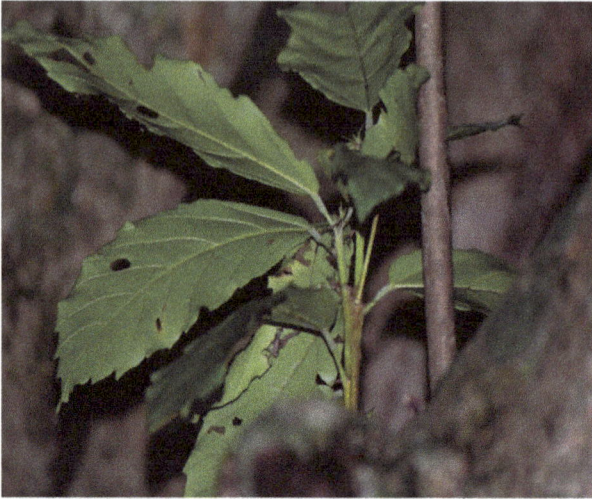

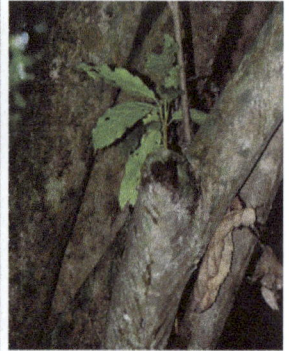

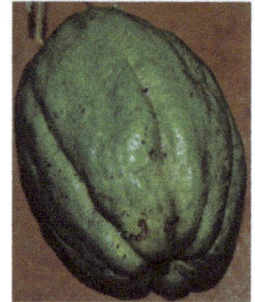

Family: Malvaceae

Botanical name: *Desplatsia dewevrei*

Common name: Elephant Okra

Local name: *Edo:* Ighiawogho, ikhubeni, *Yoruba:* Ila-erin.

Local uses: The large globose to ellipsoid and angular fibrous juicy ripe fruit of Desplatsia species are boiled to obtain a black dye used for cloth and stains like printers ink (Brink, 2009; Burkill, 2006).

Chemical constituents: The seed contains fatty acid (Hexadecanoic acid, Octadecadienoic acid; Octadecenoic acid).

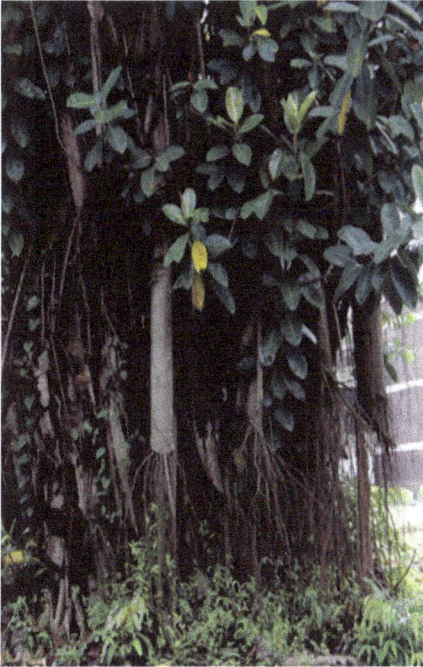

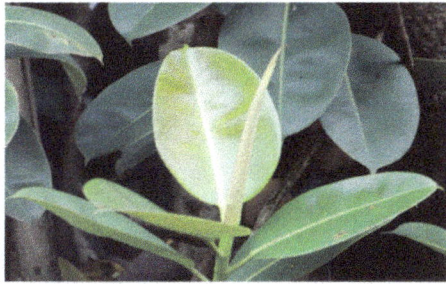

Family: Moraceae

Botanical name: *Ficus elastica*

Common name: rubber fig, rubber bush, rubber tree, rubber plant, or Indian rubber bush, Indian rubber tree.

History: *Ficus elastica*, is a species of plant in the fig genus, native to East India, Nepal, Bhutan, Burma, China (Yunnan), Malaysia, and Indonesia. It has become naturalized in Sri Lanka, the West Indies, and the United State of Florida.

Local uses: For healing wounds, cuts and bruises (Zhengyi Wu *et al.,* 2013).

Chemical constituents: Ficus elastic acid, lauric acid, myristic acid, butyric acid. The latex is used for rubber making (Chang et al.1998)

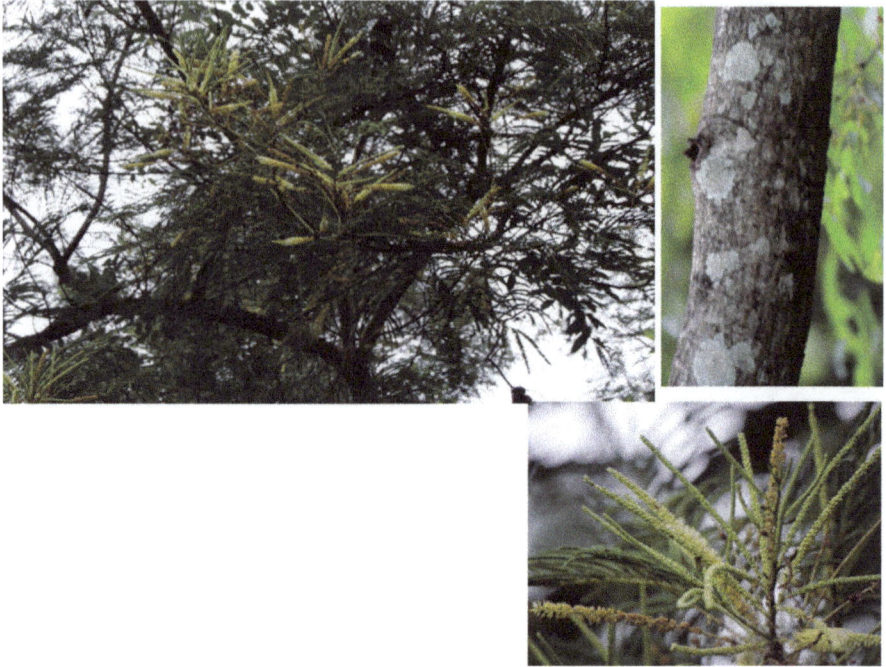

Family: Fabiaceae

Botanical name: *Entada africana*

Local name: Yoruba: Agurobe, igba oyibo, ogurobe

History: Originates from south Sahel and Sudanian ecozone savannas in disturbed places, fairly common and gregarious. Throughout the Sahel to East and South Africa.

Local uses: Tender young leaves cooked, occasionally harvested from the wild and used in sauces. The plant is commonly used as a traditional medicine within its native range. The leaves have been shown to contain retinol, the leaves are stomachic. They are used to make a tonic tea applied externally, the leaves are used for healing wounds. They make a good wound dressing, preventing suppuration. The bark is abortifacient, the roots are stimulant and tonic. Because of their emetic properties, they are said to have antidotal effects against various toxic agents and food poison. A fibre obtained from the inner bark is used for making ropes, bands, storage bins. The bark is a source of tannins. A low-quality gum is obtained from the tree. The bark contains rotenone, which has insecticidal properties (Aubréville 1950; Berhaut 1975; Geerling 1982; Von Maydell, 1983).

Chemical constituents: Tannin, saponin and rotenol (Burkill, 1995).

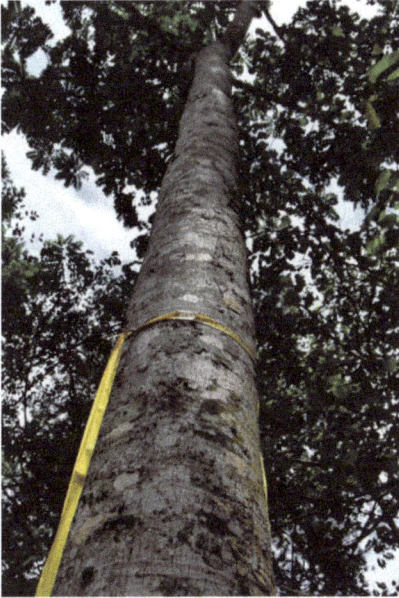

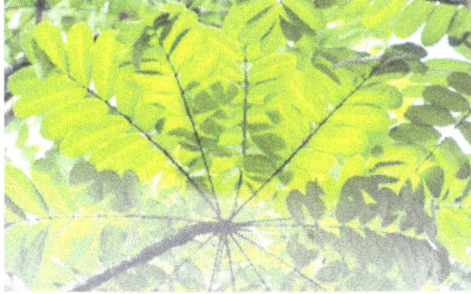

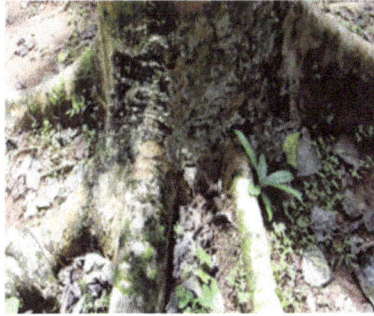

Family: Meliaceae

Botanical name: *Entandrophragma angolense*

Common name: English mountain mahogany, tiama mahogany, Tiama, acajou tiama

Local name: *Edo:* Gedunohor, *Igbo:* Okeone, *Yoruba:* Ijebo

History: *Entandrophragma angolense* is widespread, occurring from Guinea east to southern Sudan, Uganda and western Kenya, and south to DR Congo and Angola.

Local uses: The wood, usually traded as 'gedu nohor' or 'tiama', is highly valued for exterior and interior joinery, furniture, cabinet work, veneer and plywood, and is also used for flooring, interior trim, panelling, stairs, ship building, vehicle bodies and coffins. It is suitable for light construction, musical instruments, toys, novelties, boxes, crates, carvings and turnery. Wood that is not suitable as timber is used as firewood and for charcoal production. The bark is used in traditional medicine. A decoction is drunk to treat fever and the bark is also used, usually in external applications, as an anodyne against stomach-ache and peptic ulcers, earache, and kidney, rheumatic or arthritic pains. It is also applied externally to treat ophthalmia, swellings and ulcers.

The tree is planted as a roadside tree, and occasionally as a shade tree in banana, coffee and tea plantations. (Burkill, 1985; Abbiw, 1990).

Chemical constituents: Tannins, alkaloids, saponin and cardiac glycoside (Shittu and Akor, 2015).

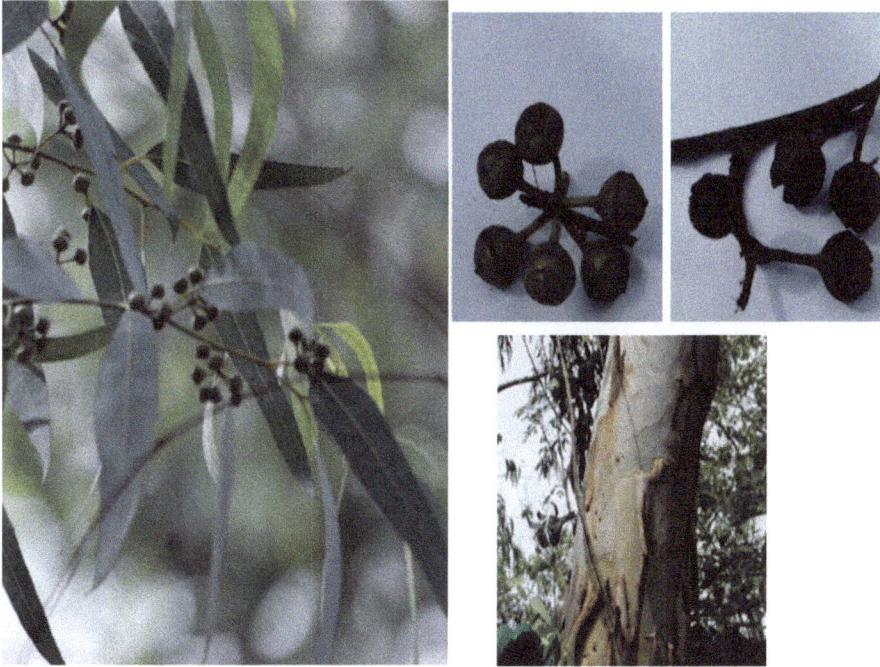

Family: Myrtaceae.

Botanical name: *Eucalyptus officinalis*

Common names: Gum trees

History: Members of the genus Eucalyptus, dominate the tree flora of Australia, and include *Eucalyptus regnans*, the tallest known flowering plant on Earth. There are more than 700 species of eucalyptus and most are native to Australia; a very small number are found in adjacent areas of New Guinea and Indonesia.

Belief: It is commonly believed that the thirst of the Eucalyptus dries up rivers and wells.

Local uses: Eucalyptus is a fast-growing evergreen tree native to Australia. As an ingredient in many over-the-counter (OTC) products, it is used to reduce symptoms of coughs, colds, and congestion. It also features in creams and ointments aimed at relieving muscle and joint pain. The oil that comes from the eucalyptus tree is used as an antiseptic, a perfume, as an ingredient in cosmetics, as a flavoring, in dental preparations, and in industrial solvents (Sadlon and Lamson, 2010).

Chemical constituents: Eucalyptol, the leaves also contain flavonoids and tannins (Low et al., 1974; Nagpal *et al.,* 2010).

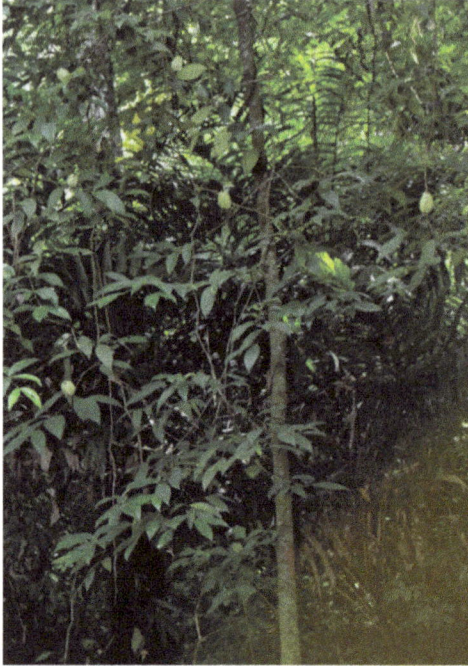

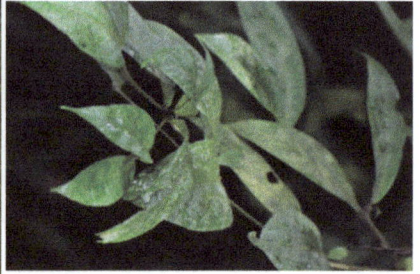

Family: Rubiaceae

Botanical name: *Rothmannia hispida*

Local name: *Edo:* Asun, asun-nekwe, asun leghere. *Yoruba:* Asogbodun

History: A shrub or small tree to 10m high; of the forest under storey, or in secondary jungle; from Guinea to W. Cameroons, and on into Zaïre. The wood on cutting and exposure to the air takes on a blue colour.

Local uses: In Nigeria, leaf sap and fruit juice are used to draw black designs on the body and to blacken tattoos; mixed with palm oil, they are applied on the skin against fungal infections (Abbiw, 1990).

Chemical constituents: Monomethyl fumarate, D-mannitol, 4-oxoni-cotinamide-1-(1'-β-D-ribofuranoside) (Abbiw, 1990).

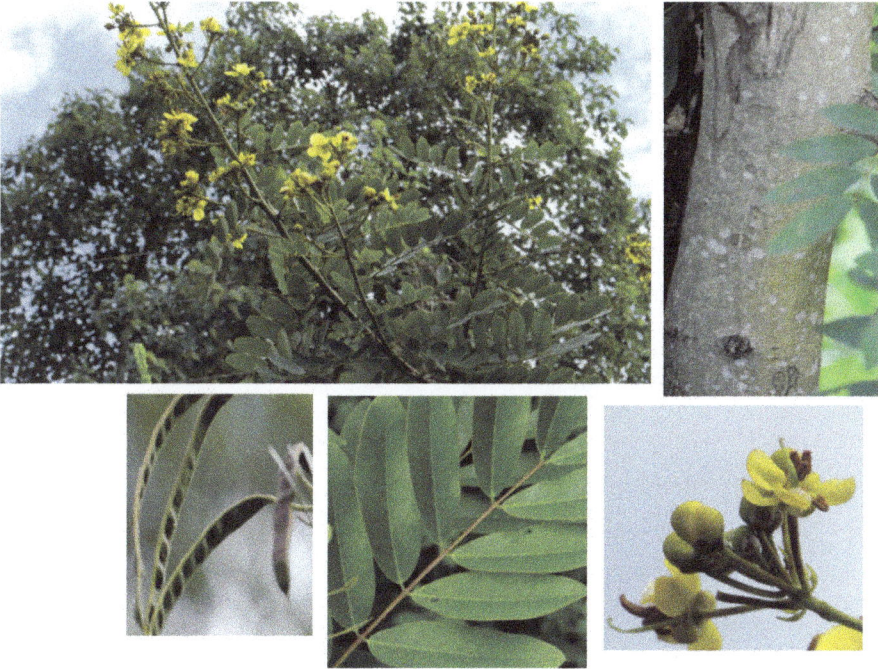

Family: Fabaceae

Botanical name: *Senna semea*

Common name: Yellow cassia, Siamese cassia, kassod tree, cassod tree and Cassia tree

History: It is native to South and Southeast Asia, although its exact origin is unknown.

Parts used: Flower, Root, Bark, Heart wood

Local uses: (flower) Food: general (root and heart-wood) Medicines: stomach troubles, venereal diseases, (heart-wood, bark, leaf, fruit, Agrihorticulture: ornamental, cultivated or partially tended Agri-horticulture: hedges, markers Agri-horticulture: biotically active Agri-horticulture: shade-trees Products: Building materials (heart-wood).

Chemical constituents: Alkaloids, saponin, phytate, anthra-quinones, oxalate, tannins and phlobatanins (Trease and Evans, 1978; Wheeler and Ferrell 1971; Day and Ununderword 1986).

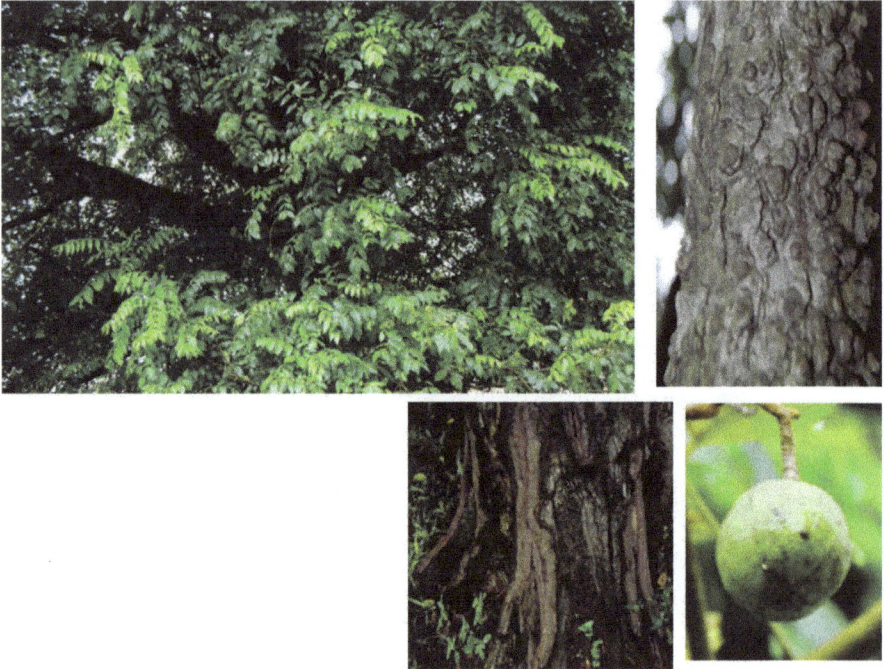

Family: Anarcadiaceae

Botanical name: *Spondias mombin*

Common name: Yellow mombin, hog plum, mombin

Local name: *Edo:* Ogheghe, okhukan, *Igbo*: Isikala, Isikere, *Yoruba*: Akika, Okikan.

History: It is native to the tropical Americas, including the West Indies. The tree has been naturalized in parts of Africa, India, Bangladesh, Sri Lanka and Indonesia. It is rarely cultivated except in parts of the Brazilian Northeast.

Local uses: The juice of crushed leaves and the powder of dried leaves are used as poultices on wounds and inflammations. The gum is employed as an expectorant and to expel tapeworms (Rodrignes and Hesse, 2000; Rodrigne and Samuels, 1999; Corthout *et al.,* 1994; Sierra and Buchelli, 1986; Ajao and Shonukan, 1985; Morton, 1987).

Chemical constituents: Anthraquinones, berberine, flavonoids, naphthoquinones, sesquiterpenes, quassiniods, indole and quinoline alkaloids (Caraballo *et al.,* 2004).

Family: Bignoniaceae

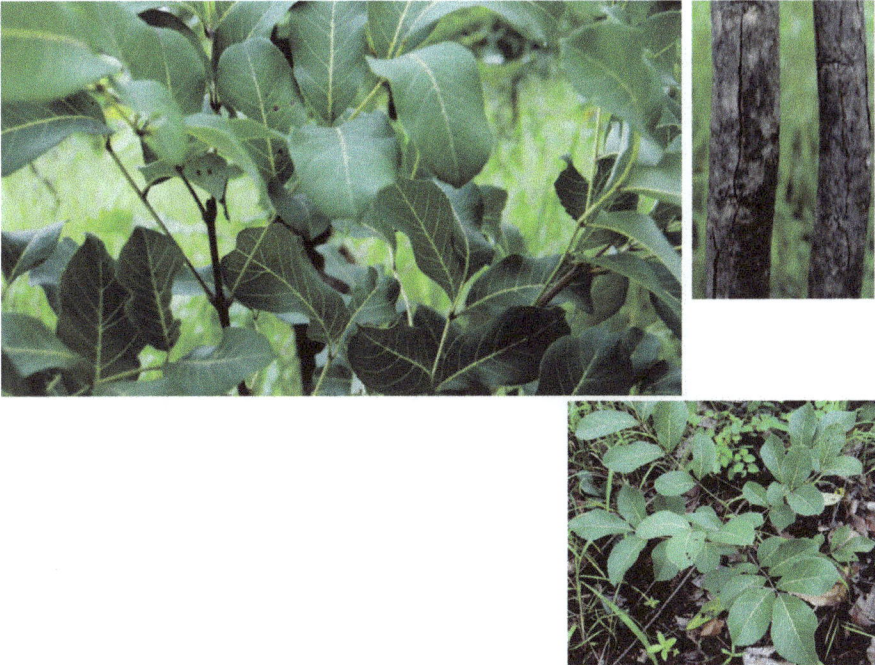

Botanical name: Stereospermum kunthianum

Local name: *Hausa*: Sansami

History: It is an African deciduous shrub or small tree occurring in the Democratic Republic of Congo, Djibouti, Eritrea, Ethiopia, Kenya, Malawi, Senegal, Somalia, Sudan, Tanzania and Uganda. It is widespread across Africa to the Red Sea, and reaches as far south as Angola, Mozambique, Zambia and Zimbabwe. There are some 30 species with a Central African and Asian distribution.

Belief: In Zaria Nigeria, the fruit is sold in local markets for magical uses. It is regarded as charm to secure riches and to woo wealthy customers.

Local uses: The pods are chewed with salt to treat coughs and are used in treatment of ulcers, leprosy, skin eruptions and venereal diseases, while the stem bark decoction or infusion is used to cure bronchitis, pneumonia, coughs, rheumatic arthritis and dysentery. The twigs are chewed to clean teeth and to treat toothache. The roots and leaves are used against venereal diseases, respiratory diseases and gastritis (Orwa *et al.,* 2009).

Chemical constituents: The phytochemical screening of the powdered stem bark revealed the presence of alkaloids, tannins, phlobatannins, saponins, cardiac glycosides, anthracene derivatives and reducing sugars (Fidelis *et al.,* 2009).

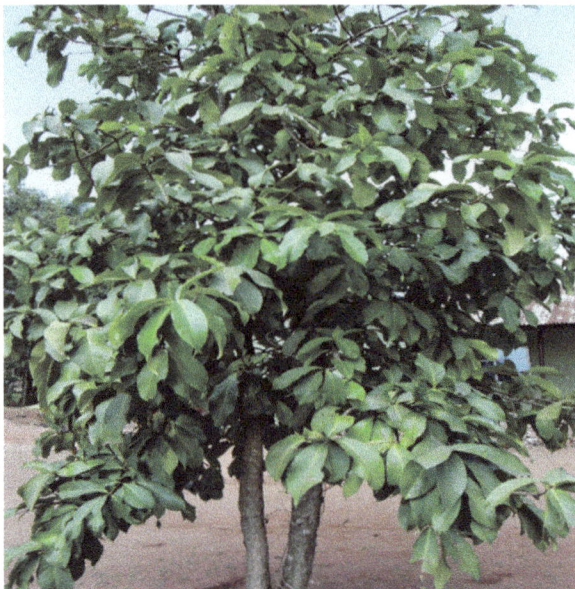

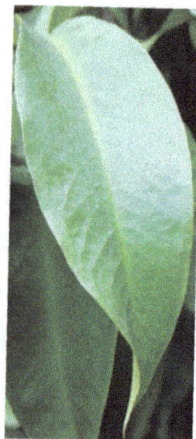

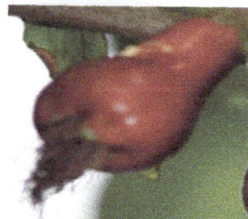

Family: Myrtaceae

Botanical name: *Syzygium samarangense*

Common name: Java apple, Semarang rose-apple and wax jambu

History: It is native to an area that includes the Greater Sunda Islands, Malay Peninsula and the Andaman and Nicobar Islands, but introduced in prehistoric times to a wider area and now widely cultivated in the tropics.

Local uses: The flowers are astringent and used in Taiwan to treat fever and halt diarrhoea.

A root-bark decoction used for dysentery abortifcacient and amenorrhea.

Powdered leaves used for cracked tongues. In Hawaii, juice of salted pounded bark used for wounds. In Molucca, decoction of bark used for thrush.

Chemical constituents: Reynoutrin, hyperin, myricitrin, quercitrin, quercetin, and guaijaverin

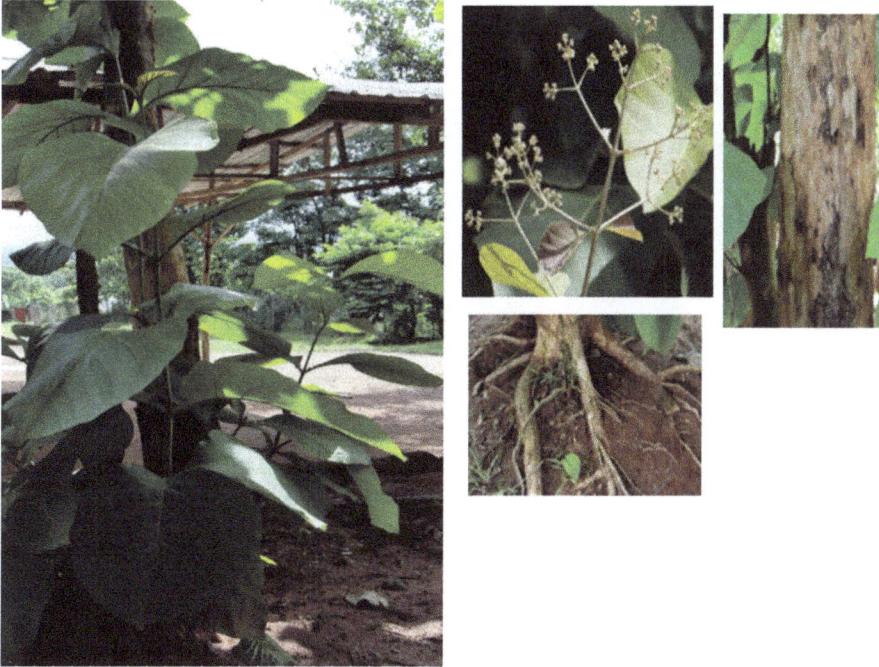

Family: Verbanaceae

Botanical name: Tectona grandis

Common name: Teak

History: *Tectona grandis* is native to south and southeast Asia, mainly India, Sri Lanka, Indonesia, Malaysia, Thailand, Myanmar and Bangladesh but is naturalised and cultivated in many countries in Africa and the Caribbean.

Local uses: It is used in the manufacture of outdoor furniture and boat decks. It is also used for cutting boards, indoor flooring, counter-tops and as a veneer for indoor furnishings. Leaves of the teak wood tree are used in making Pellakai gatti (jackfruit dumpling), where batter is poured into a teak leaf and is steamed.

Chemical constituents: Seeds contain a fixed oil containing chiefly stearic, palmitic, oleic and linoleic acids (Ghani, 2003). Root contain lapachol, tectol, dehydrotectol, tectoquinone, β-lapachone, dehydro-αlapachone and β-sitosterol (Rastogi & Mehrotra, 1993).

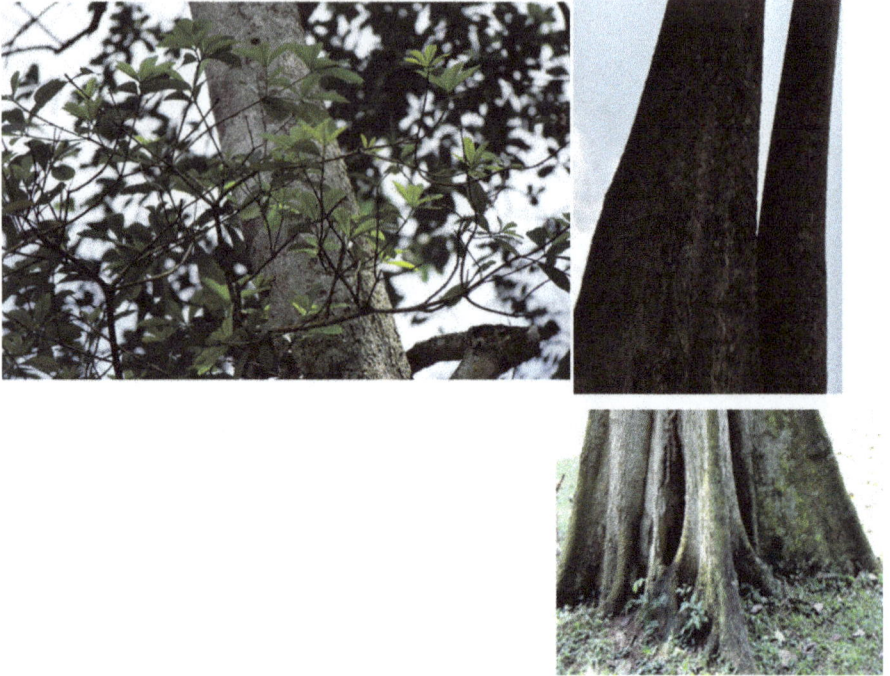

Family: Combretaceae

Botanical name: *Terminalia superba*

Common name: Shringlewood, white afara

Local name: *Edo:* Egoyen, egboin nofua, aghoin, *Yoruba*: afara

History: The family Combretaceae is comprised of 20 genera and about 475 species (Thiombiano et al.2006). Of these about 200 belong to the genus Terminalia, making it the second largest genus of the family after Combretum (McGaw *et al.,* 2001). The family is distributed throughout the tropical and sub-tropical regions of the world (Lamb and Ntima 1971). Approximately 54 species of Terminalia are naturally distributed throughout western, eastern and southern Africa (Lebrun and Stork 1991; Smith *et al.,* 2004).

Local uses: *Terminalia spp.* provide economical, medicinal, spiritual and social benefits. The wood of Terminalia spp. is highly appreciated as constructional timber. It is currently used for light construction, door and window frames, coffin boards, mouldings, beams, rafters, joists, flooring, furniture, carts, tool handles, spindles, shuttles, picker sticks, walking sticks, bowls, boat building, masts, mine props, foundation piles, veneer and plywood (Irvine 1961; Lemmens *et al.,* 1995; Schmidt *et al.,* 2002; Smith *et al.,* 2004).

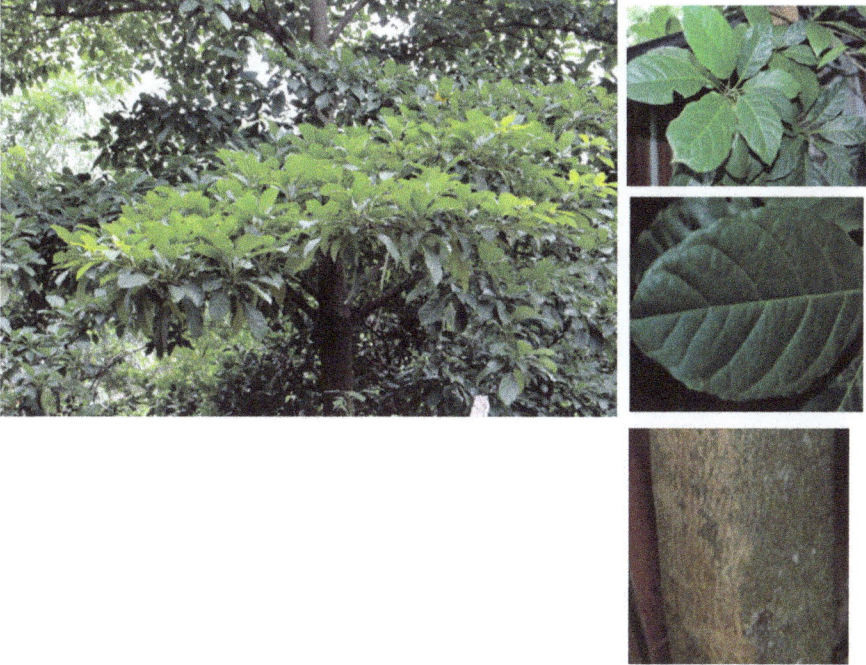

Family: Combretaceae

Botanical name: *Terminalia ivorensis*

Common name: Black afara, framire

Local name: *Edo:* ẹghọẹn-nébì, *Igbo:* awunshin-oji, *Yoruba:* Afara dudu.

History: It is found in Cameroon, Ivory Coast, Ghana, Guinea, Liberia, Nigeria, and Sierra Leone.

Local uses: The wood, usually traded as 'framiré' or 'idigbo', is valued for light construction, door and window frames, joinery, furniture, cabinet work, veneer and plywood. It is suitable for flooring, interior trim, vehicle bodies, sporting goods, boxes, crates, matches, turnery, hardboard, particle board and pulpwood. It is used locally for house construction, planks, roof shingles, fencing posts, dug-out canoes, drums and mortars. Mixed with other woods, it is suitable for paper making. The wood is also used as fire-wood and for charcoal production; offcuts are highly valued in Ghana for making charcoal.

Chemical constituents: Nitrogen, calcium and magnesium.

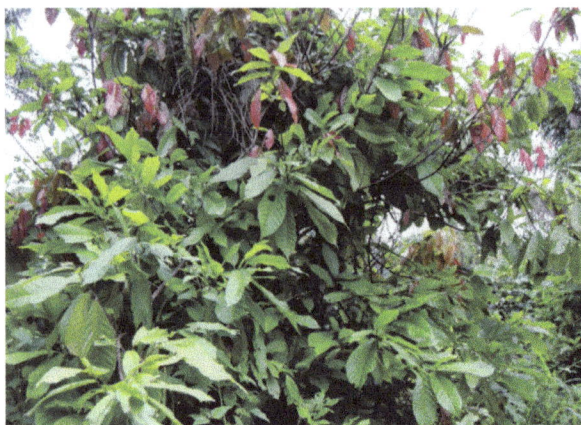

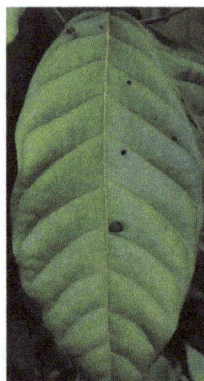

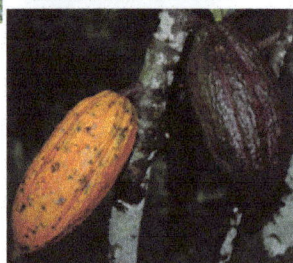

Family: Malvaceae

Botanical name: *Theombroma cacao*

Common name: Cocoa

Local name: *Edo:* Koko. *Igbo*: Koko. *Hausa*: koko *Yoruba*: koko

History: Native to the deep tropical regions of Central and South America.

Belief: The Maya believed the kakaw (cacao) was discovered by the gods in a mountain that also contained other delectable foods to be used by them. According to Maya mythology, the Plumed Serpent gave cacao to the Maya after humans were created from maize by divine grandmother goddess Xmucane. The Maya celebrated an annual festival in April to honor their cacao god, Ek Chuah, an event that included the sacrifice of a dog with cacao-colored markings, additional animal sacrifices, offerings of cacao, feathers and incense, and an exchange of gifts. (Bogin 1997, Coe 1996, Montejo 1999, Tedlock 1985).

Local uses: Its seeds and cocoa beans, are used to make cocoa mass, powder, confectionery, ganache and chocolate.

Chemical constituents: Theobromine, alkaloids, flavanals, proanthocyanidins and pectin (Decroix *et al.,* 2016).

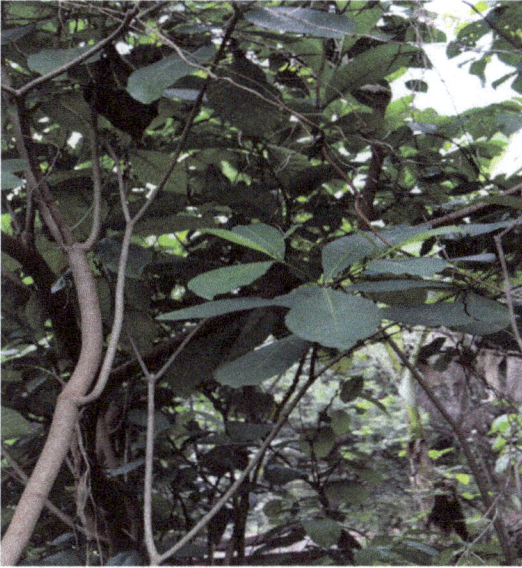

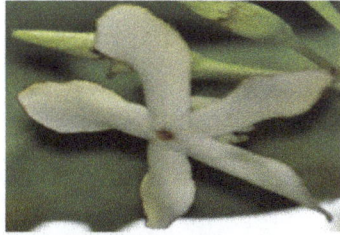

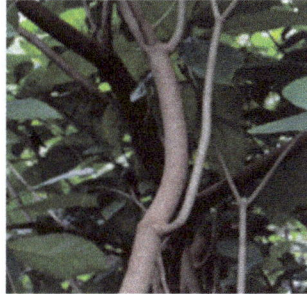

Family: Apocynaceae

Botanical name: *Voacanga africana*

Common name: Catapult plant

Local name: *Edo:* Òvìẹn-íbù. *Igbo*: Pete pete, akẹte. *Yoruba*: Akọ dodo. *Hausa:* kookiyar birii

History: *Voacanga africana* is a small tropical African tree that grows to 6m in height. It has leaves that are up to 30 cm in length, and the tree produces yellow or white flowers, which become berries with yellow seeds.

Local uses: The bark and seeds of the tree are used in Ghana as a poison, stimulant and aphrodisiac. The milky latex of the plant is applied to wounds in Nigeria and Senegal. Tea made from the leaves is said to be a strengthening potion that relieves fatigue and shortness of breath. It is also used to prevent premature childbirth and to treat painful hernias and menstruation. It is used in many areas of Africa to treat heart troubles. The seeds of *Voacanga spp.* are used in Europe due to their high tabersonine content. This is used as a precursor for vincamine, which is used to treat neural deficiencies in the elderly (Vooglebreinder 2009, 349).

Chemical constituents: Iboga alkaloids such as voacangine, voacamine, vobtusine, amataine, akuammidine, tabersonine, coronaridine and vocangine.

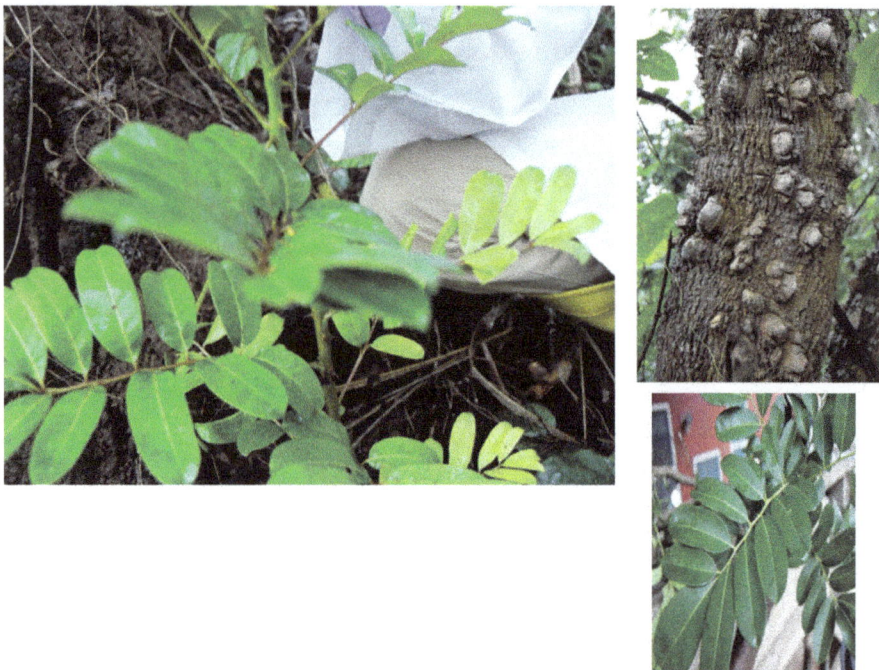

Family: Rutaceae

Botanical name: *Zanthoxylum zanthoxyloides*

Common name: Fagara

Local Names: *Edo:* Ughanghan, *Hausa*: Fasa kwari. *Igbo:* Uko. *Yoruba*: Ata

History: It occurs predominantly in Africa from Guinea east to Ghana.

Local uses: In southern Nigeria a decoction of the stem bark and roots is taken to treat cancer. Pulped stem bark and root bark is thrown in the water to stupefy fish. In West Africa, it is planted as a hedge, as the thorns make it impenetrable. Sheep browse the leaves. The wood is used for manufacturing of torches. The timber is yellow, very hard and termite-resistant and used for building purposes, including poles and posts. It also makes good firewood. The roots, young shoots and twigs are commonly used as chewsticks. The bark or young branches contain much resin, which makes them suitable for ceremonial torches. The spines are thrown into fire to give off a scented smoke. The leaves, which smell like citronella, and the seeds, which taste strongly of cinnamon or pepper, are commonly used to season food. From the seeds, necklaces are made.

Zanthoxyloides is believed to also have numerous magico-religious uses, including protection against spirits. It also serves as fetish plant (Arbonier, 2004). 70

Chemical Constituents: Acridone alkaloids, namely, 3-hydroxy- 1 ,5 ,6 - t r imethoxy- 9 -acridone;1 ,6 - dihydroxy- 3- methoxy- 9 - acridone; 3,4,5,7-tetrahydroxy-1- methoxy-10-methyl-9- acridone; 4-methoxyzan-thacridone; (Wouatsa *et al.,* 2013)

Location: Ewu

References

Abbiw, D. (1990). Useful Plants of Ghana: West African Uses of Wild and Cultivated Plants, Intermediate Technology Publications, Royal Botanic Gardens, Kew, Richmond, United Kingdom. 337 pp.

Agbor AG, Ngogang YJ. Toxicity of herbal preparations. Cam J Ethnobot. 2005; 1:23–28.

Aguzue, Onyinye Chinelo., Akanji, Fausat Temilola, Tafida., Muazu Abubakar. Kamal, Muhammed Jamal and Abdulahi, Surajo Habibu (2012,). Comparative chemical constituents of some desert fruits in Northern Nigeria. Applied science Research 4 (2):1061-1064.

Ahsan MR, Islam KM, Bulbul IJ, Musaddik MA, Haque ME (2009). Hepatoprotective activity of methanol extract of some medicinal plants against carbon tetrachloride-induced hepatotoxicity in rats. Eur J Sci Res. 37:302–310.

Ahsan MR, Islam KM, Haque ME, Mossaddik MA (2009). In vitro antimicrobial screening and toxicity study of some different medicinal plants. Wolrd J Agri Sci. 5:617–621.

Aibinu I, Adenipekun T, Adelowotan T, Ogunsanya T, Odugbemi T (2006). Evaluation of the antimicrobial properties of different parts of Citrus aurantifolia (lime fruit) as used locally. Afr J Tradit Complement Altern Med, 4:185–90.

Ajibesin K.K. 2011. Dacryodes edulis (G. Don) H.J. Lam: A review on its medicinal, phytochemical and economical properties. Research Journal of Medicinal Plant 5(1):32-41.

Aké Assi, L., Abeye, J., Guinko, S., Riguet, R. & Bangavou, X., 1985. Médecine traditionnelle et pharmacopée - Contribution aux tudes ethnobotaniques et floristiques en République Centrafricaine. Agence de Coopération Culturelle et Technique, Paris, France. 140 pp.

Antimicrobial and antimalarial activity of Cussonia species (Araliaceae). Journal of Ethnopharmacology 129: 189-196.

Aubréville A. (1950). Flore forestière Soudano-Guinéenne, AOF, Cameroun, AEF. Soc. Ed. Géogr. Marit. & Colon., Paris. 523pp

Bailey, L.H. & E.Z. Bailey. 1976. Hortus Third i–xiv, 1–1290. Collier & Son Company. MacMillan, New York.

Beentje, H.J., 1994. Kenya trees, shrubs and lianas. National Museums of Kenya, Nairobi, Kenya. 722 pp. erhaut J. (1975). Flore illustrée du

Sénégal. vol. 4: Ficoïdées à Légumineuses. Direction des Eaux et Forêts, Ministère du Développement Rural, Dakar. 525 pp

Berhow MA, Bennett RD, Poling SM, Vannier S, Hidaka T, Omura M (1994). Acylated flavonoids in callus cultures of Citrus aurantifolia. Phytochemistry.36:1225–7.

Bisset, N.G. "Phytochemistry and Pharmacology of Voacanga Species." Agricultural University Wageningen Papers 85, no. 3 (1985):81–114.

Boland, D. J.; Brooker, M. I. H.; Chippendale, G. M.; McDonald, M. W. (2006). Forest trees of Australia (5th ed.). Collingwood, Vic.: CSIRO Publishing. p. 82.

Botanical Garden, St. Louis, MO & Harvard University Herbaria, Cambridge, MA. Retrieved 29 August 2013.

Bringmann, G., Hamm, A., Kraus, J., Ochse, M., Noureldeen, A. & Jumbam, D.N., 2001. Gardenamide A from Rothmannia urcelliformis (Rubiaceae) - isolation, absolute stereostructure, and biomimetic synthesis from genipine. European Journal of Organic Chemistry 10: 1983–1987.

Brink, M., 2009, 'Desplatsia subericarpa Bocq', Record from PROTA4U, in M. Brink & E.G. Achigan-Dako (eds.), PROTA (Plant Resources of Tropical Africa/Ressources végétales de l'Afrique tropicale), Wageningen, Netherlands, viewed 21 July 2015, from http://www.prota4u.org/search.asp

Burkill H.M (1985). The Useful Plants of Tropical West Africa (second edition) vol.1 (Families A-D) pp. 138–140 pub. Royal Botanic Gardens, Kew.

Burkill, 1985. In: The Useful Plants of Tropical West Africa, Vol 3, Royal Botanic Gardens, Kew, UK.

Burkill, H.M. (1985). The Useful Plants of Tropical West Africa, 1: pp.211-212.

Burkill, H.M. 1985. The Useful Plants of Tropical West Africa, Vol 4.

Burkill, H.M. (2006). The Useful Plants of Tropical West Africa 1, vol. 5, 2nd edn., Royal Botanical Garden, Kew, Richmond, Surrey.

Burkill, H.M., 2000. The Useful Plants of Tropical West Africa. 2nd Edition. Volume 5, Families S–Z, Addenda. Royal Botanic Gardens, Kew, Richmond, United Kingdom. 686 pp.

C.K. Firempong, L. A. Andoh, *W. G. Akanwariwiak, P. Addo Fordjour and P. Adjakofi (2016). Phytochemical screening and antifungal activities of crude ethanol extracts of red flowered silk cotton tree (Bombax buonopozense) and Calabash nutmeg (Monodora myristica) on Candidaalbicans.Department of Biochemistry and Biotechnology, Kwame Nkrumah University of Scienceand Technology, Kumasi Ghana. Journal of Microbiology and Antimicrobials, 8(4): 22-27

Caristi C, Bellocco E, Panzera V, Toscano G, Vadalà R, Leuzzi U (2003). Flavonoids detection by HPLC-DAD-MS-MS in lemon juices from Sicilian cultivars. J Agric Food Chem., 51:3528–34.

Chang Siushih, Wu Chengyih and Cao Ziyu (1998). Moroideae. In: Chang Siushih & Wu Chengyih, eds., Fl. Reipubl. Popularis Sin. 23(1): 1–219.

Chopra, R. N., Nayer, S. L. and Chopra, I. C. (1956). Glossary of Indian Medicinal Plants, CSIR, New Delhi, 1956.

Chukwuma, O. E. (2015), Antioxidative activity of the almond leaves (Terminalia Catappa), International Journal of Nursing, Midwife and Health Related Cases Vol.1, No.2, pp.29-40.

Cooke, B; Ernst, E (2000). Aromatherapy: A systematic review. British Journal of General Practice. 50 (455): 493–6.

Corthout J., Pieters L. A., Claeys M., Vanden Berghe D. A. and Viletinck J. (1994): Antibacterial and molluscicidal phenolic acid from Spondias mombin.

Cowan, M.M., 1999. Plant products as antimicrobial agents. Clin Microbiol. Rev., 12: 564-582.

Dalziel, J.M., 1937. The useful plants of West Tropical Africa. Crown Agents for Overseas Governments and Administrations, London, United Kingdom. 612 pp.

De Villiers, B.J., Van Vuuren, S.F., Van Zyl, R.F. and Van Wyk, B.E. (2010).

Decroix, Lieselot; Tonoli, Cajsa; Soares, Danusa D.; Tagougui, Semah; Heyman, Elsa; Meeusen, Romain (2016-12-01). "Acute cocoa flavanol improves cerebral oxygenation without enhancing executive function at rest or after exercise". Applied Physiology, Nutrition, and Metabolism. 41 (12): 1225–1232.Dressler, S.; Schmidt, M. & Zizka, G. (2014).

Dialium guineense. African plants – a Photo Guide. Frankfurt/Main: Forschungsinstitut Senckenberg

Ezeokonkwo, C. A. and Dodson, W. L. (2004), The potential of Terminalia catappa (Tropical almond) seed as a source of dietary protein, Journal of Food Quality, vol. 27, issue 3, pp. 207-219.

F. Maiza-Benabdesselam, M. Chibane, K. Madani, H. Max, and S. Adach,(2007). Determination of isoquinoline alkaloids contents in two Algerian species of Fumaria (Fumaria capreolata and

Forget P. M.; et al. (2009). A new species of Carapa (Meliaceae) from Central Guyana . Brittonia. 61 (4): 366–74.

Fumaria bastardi), African Journal of Biotechnology, 6(21); 2487-2492

G. Kweio-Okai,(1991) "Antiinammatory activity of a Ghanaian antiarthritic herbal preparation: II," Journal of Ethnopharmacol- Geerling (1982). Guide de terrain des ligneux sahéliens et soudano-guinéens (2 eme éd.). Agricult. Univ., Wageningen. Grasses and Legumes Index (1st ed. 1982) 340 pp. herbpathy. com (Material Medical: How to Use Entandrophragma angolense) Accessed September, 2017

Heuzé V., Tran G., Archimède H., Bastianelli D., Lebas F., 2015. Neem (Azadirachta indica). Feedipedia, a programme by INRA, CIRAD, AFZ and FAO. https://feedipedia.org/node/182 Last updated on October 2, 2015, 15:40

Jain SK, Dam N (1979). Some ethnobotanical notes from Northeastern India. Economic Botany, 33:52–56.

Kawaii S, Tomono Y, Katase E, Ogawa K, Yano M (1999). Quantitation of flavonoid constituents in Citrus fruits. J Agric Food Chem.,47:3565–71.

Kenfack D.; Peréz A. J. (2011). Two new species of Carapa (Meliaceae) from western Ecuador. Systematic Botany. 36 (1): 124–28.

Khandelwal KR. Pune: Nirali Prakashan; 2006. Practical Pharmacognosy; p. 149.

Kiecolt-Glaser, J. K.; Graham, J. E.; Malarkey, W. B.; Porter,

K. Lemeshow, S; Glaser, R (2008). Olfactory influences on mood and autonomic, endocrine, and immune function Psychoneuroendocrinology. 33 (3): 328–39.

Low D, Rawal BD and Griffin WJ (1974). Antibacterial action of the essential oils of some Australian Myrtaceae with special references to the activity of chromatographic fractions of oil of Eucalyptus citriodora. Planta Med. 26:184-185.

Miot HA, Batistella RF, Batista Kde A, Volpato DE, Augusto LS, Madeira NG, Haddad V Jr, Miot LD (2004). Comparative study of the topical effectiveness of the Andiroba oil (Carapa guianensis) and DEET 50% as repellent for Aedes sp. Rev Inst Med Trop Sao Paulo. 46 (5): 253–6.

N. Nagpal, G. Shah, M. Arora N., R. Shri and Y. Arya (2010 PHYTO-CHEMICAL AND PHARMACOLOGICAL ASPECTS OF EU-CALYPTUS GENUS. International Journal of Pharmaceutical Sciences And Research 3:28-36 National Journal of PharmTech Research, 2(1) 18-25

National Research Council (2008). "Butterfruit". Lost Crops of Africa: Volume III: Fruits. Lost Crops of Africa. 3. National Academies Press.

Neuwinger, H.D., 2000. African traditional medicine: a dictionary of plant use and applications. Medpharm Scientific, Stuttgart, Germany. 589 pp.

Niangoran Bouah, Georges (1983). Les Aboure, une société lagunaire de Côte d'Ivoire. AUA, Lettres et Sciences Humaines 1 … AUA F,11: 5–12. Niangoran Bouah, Georges. Idéologie de l'or chez les Akan de Côte d'Ivoire et du

Nwankwo IU, Osaro-Matthew RC, Ekpe IN (2015). Synergistic antibacterial potentials of Citrus aurantifolia (Lime) and honey against some bacteria isolated from sputum of patients attending Federal Medical Center, Umuahia. Int J Curr Microbiol Appl Sci.4:534–44. ogy, 33(1-2): 129-133

Omonhinmin A Conrad and Agbara I Uche (2013). Assessment of In vivo antioxidant properties of Dacryodes edulis and Ficus exasperata as anti-malaria plants. Asian Pac J Trop Dis. 3(4): 294–300

Orwa C, Mutua A, Kindt R, Jamnadass R, Simons A. Agroforestree Database: a tree reference and selection guide version 4.0. 2009 http://www.worldagroforestry.org/af/treedb/ Oxford University Press, London.

Palanichamy, S., Nagarajan,S., and Devasagayam,M. (1998).J. Ethnopharmacol., 22: 81-90

Palunichamy, S., and Nagarajan, S. (1990). Antifungal activity of Cassia alata Linn leaf extract. J. Ethnopharmacol., 29:337-340.Pathan R, Papi R, Parveen P, Tananki G, Soujanya P (2012). In vitro antimicrobial activity of Citrus aurantifolia and its phytochemical screening. Asian Pac J Trop Dis. 2:328–31

Penniston KL, Nakada SY, Holmes RP, Assimos DG (2008) Quantitative Assessment of Citric Acid in Lemon Juice, Lime Juice, and Commercially-Available Fruit Juice Products. Journal of Endourology. 22 (3): 567–570 plantfadb.bch.msu.edu/plants_ pubs/37716. Accessed 25/9/2017

Pradeep G, Anil K A, Lakash MS and Singh GK (2015). Antidiabetic and antihyperlipidemic effect of Borassus flabellifer in streptozotocin (STZ) induced diabetic rats. World Journal of Pharmacy and Pharmaceutical Sciences 4(1):1172-1184

Rauf A, Uddin G, Ali J (2014). Phytochemical analysis and radical scavenging profile of juices of Citrus sinensis, Citrus anrantifolia, and Citrus limonum. Org Med Chem Lett. 4: 5.

Reynolds, Francis J. (1921).Deleb palm". Collier's New Encyclopedia. New York: P.F.

S dsee-Speer (2014): Hamburger Forscher bestimmt Holzart - SPIEGEL ONLINE. SPIEGEL ONLINE. 30 May 2014. Retrieved 25 September 2014.

S. Arulmozhi, P. M. Mazumder, L. S. Narayanan, and P. Akurdesai (2010). In vitro antioxidant and free radical scavenging activity of fractions from Alstonia scholaris Linn. R. Br, Inter-S. Zillur

Rahman and M. Shamim Jairajpuri (1996). Neem in Unani Medicine. Neem Research and Development Society of Pesticide Science, India, New Delhi, February 1993, p. 208-219. Edited by N.S. Randhawa and B.S. Parmar. 2nd revised edition,

Sadlon AE, Lamson DW (2010). Immune-modifying and antimicrobial effects of Eucalyptus oil and simple inhalation devices. Altern Med Rev. 15(1):33-47.

Shittu GA, and Akor ES (2015). Phytochemical screening and antimicrobial activities of the leaf extract of Entandrophragama angolense. African Journal of Biotechnology, 14:3

Thiombiano A, Schmidt M, Kreft H, Guinko S, 2006. Influence du gradient climatique sur la distribution des espèces de Combretaceae au Burkina Faso (Afrique de l'ouest). Candollea 61, 189-213.

Trease, M.T. and S.E. Evans, 1978. The phytochemical analysis and antibacterial screening of extracts of Tetracarpetum conophorum. J. Chem. Sci Nig., 26: 57-58. Wheeler. A.B. and M.D. Ferrell, 1971. The phytochemical

Utubaku AB, Yakubu OE and Okwara DU (2017). Comparative Phytochemical Analysis of Fermented and Unfermented Seeds of Dialium giuneense. Department of Medical Biochemistry, Cross River University of Technology, Calabar, Nigeria and Department of Biochemistry, Federal University Wukari, Nigeria, Journal of Traditional Medicine & Clinical Naturopathy

Von Maydell, J. (1983) Arbres et Arbustes du Sahel, leurs caractéristiques et leurs utilisations. Publié par GTZ, Hambourg, 310 p.

Voogelbreinder, Snu, Garden of Eden: The Shamanic Use of sychoactive Flora and Fauna, and the Study of Consciousness. Snu Voogelbreinder, 2009.

Wouatsa, V.N. et al., 2013. Aromatase and glycosyl transferase inhibiting acridone alkaloids from fruits of Cameroonian Zanthoxylum species. Chemistry Central journal, 7(1), p.125.

Yenon Achiè Aurélie, Koffi Akissi Jeanne, Bedou Kouassi Denis, Yapi Houphouet Félix, Nguessan Jean David and Djaman Allico Joseph (2017). Anti-inflammatory Effect of Entandrophragma angolense Bark Extracts on Acute Edema of the Rat's Paw Induced by Carrageenan. International Journal of Biochemistry Research & Review, 18 (3). ISSN: 2231-086X.

Zhengyi Wu, Zhe-Kun Zhou & Michael G. Gilbert. Ficus elastica. Flora of China. Missouri

Chapter 4

Shrubs

This chapter looks at some common and uncommon shrubs which are used traditionally to solve both physical and spiritual health problems in local communities in Nigeria and Africa. Shrubs refer to plants that are smaller than trees, usually having several stems rather than a single trunk.

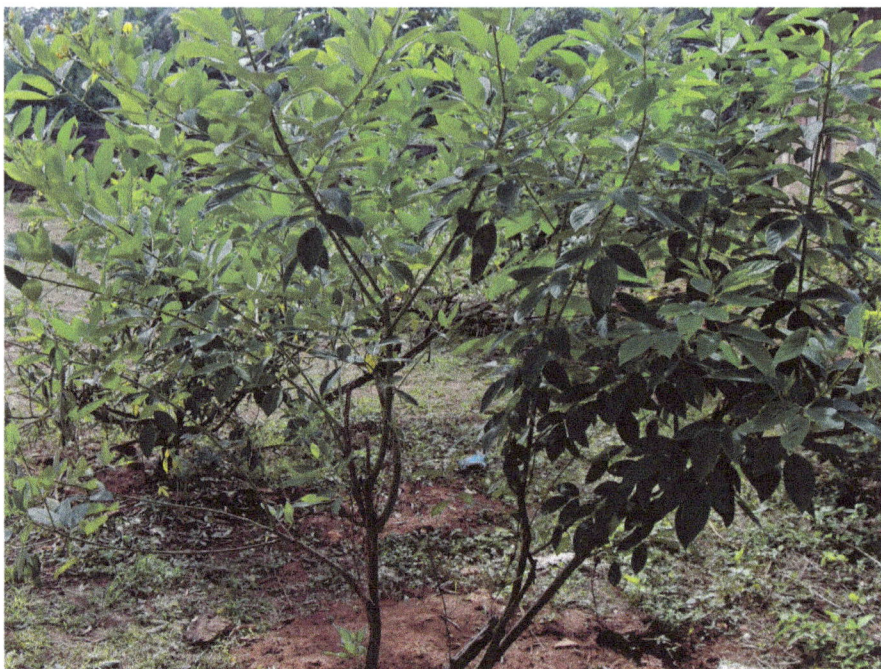

Family: Fabaceae

Botanical name: *Cajanus cajan*

Common names: Pigeon pea

Local names: *Edo:* Olele. *Hausa:* Waaken tantabara, Dan-mata. *Igbo:* Fio-fio. *Yoruba:* Otili

History: *Cajanus cajan*, more commonly known as pigeon pea, is a drought-resistant crop important for small scale farmers in semi-arid areas where rainfall is low. Probably native to India, pigeon pea was brought millennia ago to Africa where different strains developed. These were brought to the new world in post-Columbian times. Truly wild Cajanus has never been found; they exist mostly as remnants of cultivation.

Parts used: Leaves and Seeds

Local Uses: In India and Java, the young leaves are applied to sores. The Indo-chinese claim that powdered leaves help expel bladderstones. Salted leaf juice is taken for jaundice. In Argentina the leaf decoction is prized for genital and other skin irritations, especially in females. Floral decoctions are used for bronchitis, coughs, and pneumonia. Chinese shops sell dried roots as an alexeritic, anthelminthic, expectorant, sedative, and vulnerary. Leaves are also used for toothache, mouthwash, sore gums, child-delivery, dysentery. Scorched seed, added to coffee, are said to alleviate headache and vertigo. Fresh seeds are said to help incontinence of urine in males, while immature fruits are believed of use in liver and kidney. In recent years it has also been explored for the treatment of ischemic necrosis of the caput femoris, aphtha, bedsore and wound healing (Yuan-gang *et al.,* 2010).

Chemical constituents: Cajanin, concajanin, methionine, lysine, and tryptophan (Bressani *et al.,* 1986)

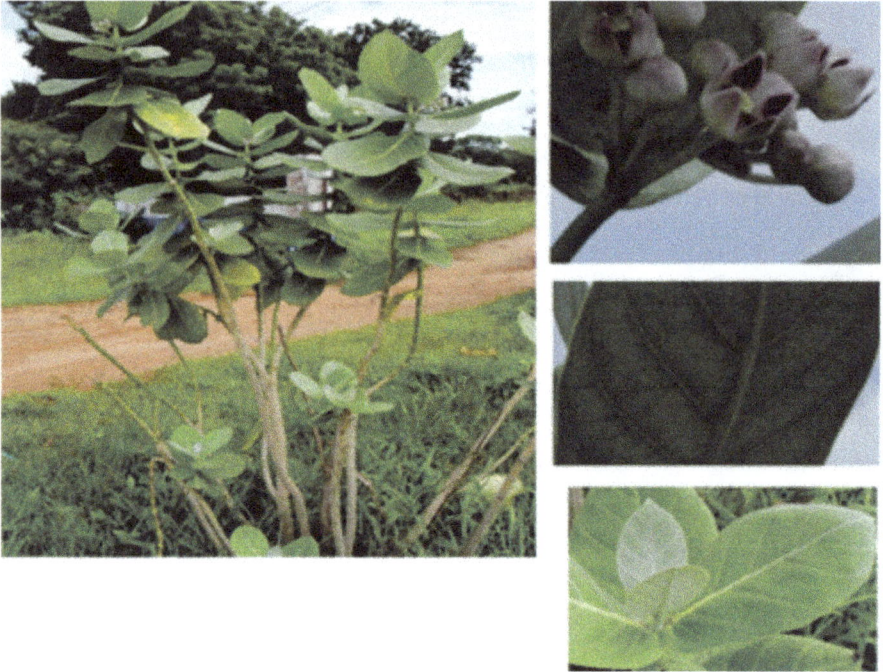

Family: Asclepiadaceae

Botanical name: *Calotropis Procera*

Common names: Giant milk weed, Soddom apple

Local name: *Hausa*: Baabaa ambalee, *Igbo*: Otokwuru. *Yoruba*: Bomubomu

History: The fruit is described by the Roman Jewish historian Josephus, who saw it growing near Sodom; "as well as the ashes growing in their fruits; which fruits have a color as if they were fit to be eaten, but if you pluck them with your hands, they dissolve into smoke and ashes."

Belief: Some biblical commentators believe that the Sodom Apple may have been the poisonous gourd (or poison-tasting gourd) that led to "death in the pot" in 2 Kings 4:38–41.

Parts used: Leaves, root, bark, latex

Local uses: *Calotropis procera* latex has been used in leprosy, eczema, inflammation, cutaneous infections, syphilis, malarial and low hectic fevers, and as abortifacient (Kumar and Basu, 1994; Sharma and Sharma, 2000).

Chemical constituents: Calotropin, Calotoxin, Resinols, alkaloids, flavonoids, tannins, Saponins, and Cardiac glycosides (Mainasara *et al.,* 2011).

Location: Afasho

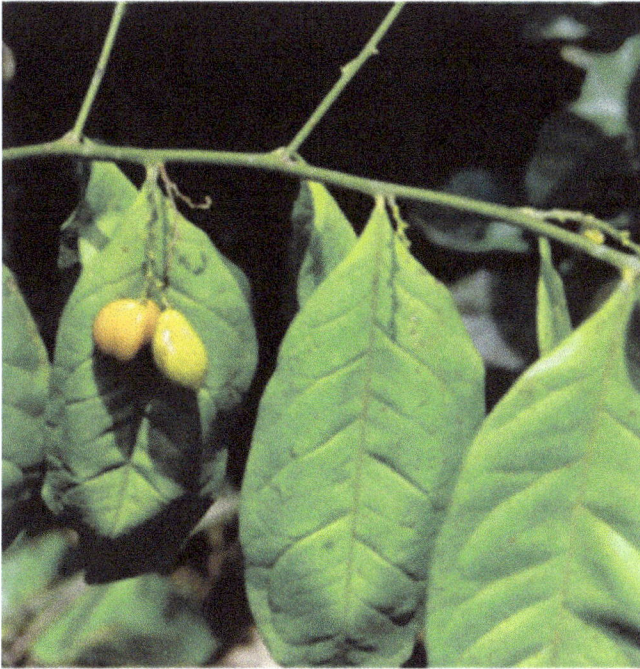

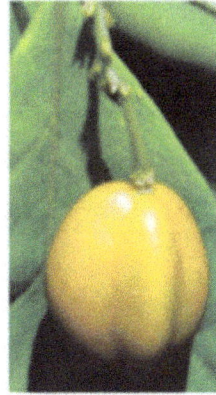

Family: Polygalaceae

Botanical name: *Carpolobia lutea*

Common name: Cattlestick

Local name: *Edo:* Aswen. *Igbo*: Aghba-awa. *Yoruba*: Amurejo

History: It is widely distributed in West and Central areas of tropical Africa.

Local Uses: The stem is used as chewing stick, the root is also used as chewing stick because of its aphrodisiac potentials. Its shrubby and smallish stems give it a ornamental use as sweeping material or broom in rural areas among the Ibibio tribes of Akwa Ibom State, Nigeria. The resilience of the woody stem enhances its patronage by cattle herders as cane to control their cattle heads. The decoction of the root is used in locally-made alcohol as an aphrodisiac. It is used in the treatment of genitourinary infections, gingivitis and waist pains (Ettebong and Nwafor, 2009).

Chemical Constituents: Triterpene saponins and polyphenol (Nwidu, 2010)

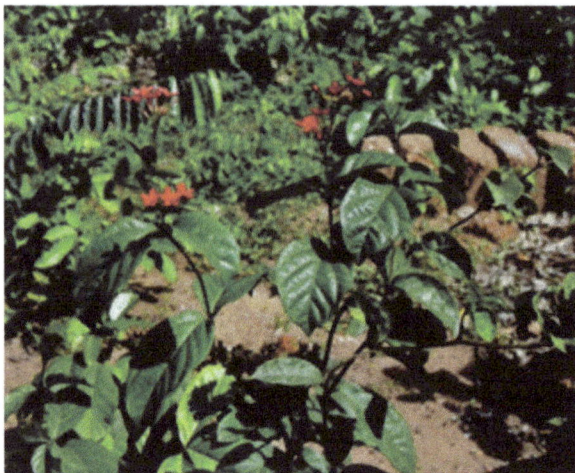

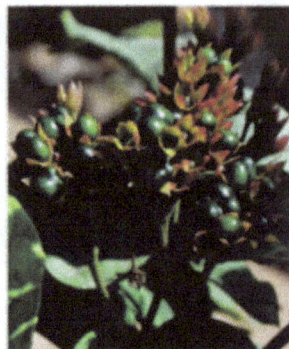

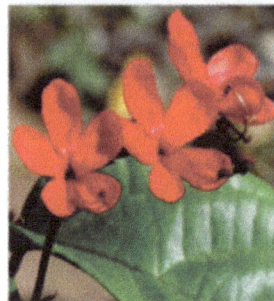

Family: Lamiaceae

Botanical name: *Clerodendrum splendens*

Common name: Flaming glory bower, glory tree

Local name: *Igbo*: Afifia omya, Ufuchi, *Yoruba*: Adabi, Opo-eshi, Araojola

History: It is a native of tropical West Africa.

Local uses: The plant is used ethnomedicinally in Ghana for the treatment of vaginal thrush, bruises, wounds and various skin infections (Irvine, 1961).

Chemical Constituents: Carbohydrates, glycosides, unsaturated sterols, triterpenoids and flavonoids are reported to be present in the leaves, in addition to volatile oil in the flowers (Shehata *et al.,* 2001 and el-Deeb, 2003)

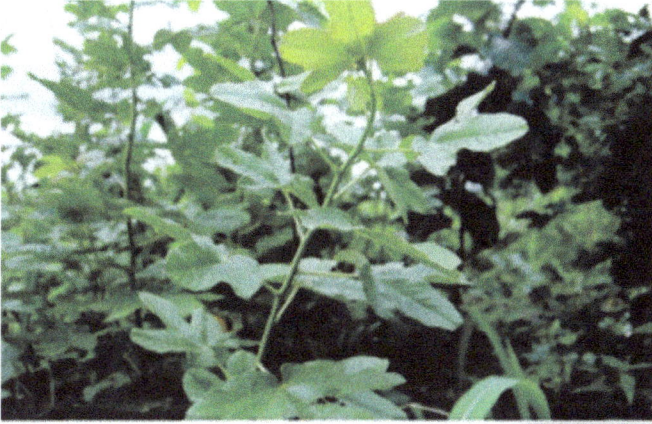

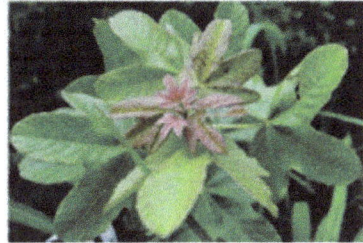

Family: Cochlospermaceae

Botanical name: *Cochlospermum planchonii*

Common name: False cotton

Local name: *Edo:* Gbutu. *Hausa:* Zunzunaa. *Yoruba:* Oboyo

History: It originates in western tropical Africa, from Senegal to Sierra Leone, east to Chad and northern Cameroon.

Belief: The Fulani of Northern Nigeria believe that a leaf-infusion bestows magical protection.

Local uses: The root is a source of a yellow dye which is used in Sudan and in Nupe and elsewhere. Hausas in Northern Nigeria add indigo to obtain green shades. The root is used in Lagos in cooking soup when oil is not available. This explains the anti-diarrhoeal use of *C. planchonii* root in traditional medicine. In addition, the tannin has astringent properties, hastens the healing of wounds and inflamed mucous membrane. Plants with tannins are used for healing of wounds, hemorrhoids and diabetes (Yakubu et al., 2010: Salah *et al.,* 1995).

Chemical constituents: *phytochemicals,* Prominent among which are saponins, alkaloids, phenolics and steroids (Mikhail and Musbau, 2013).

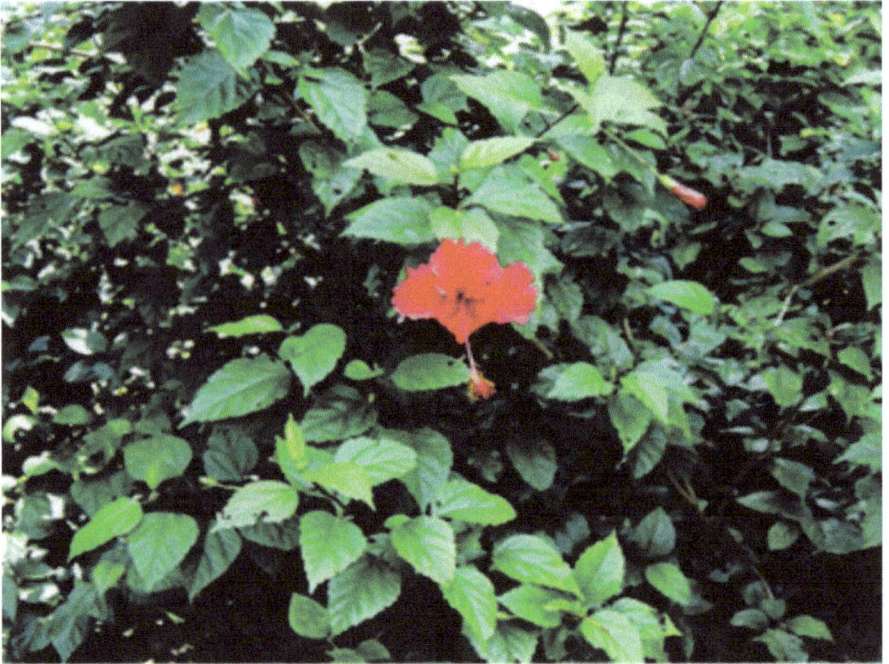

Family: Malvaceae

Botanical name: *Hibiscus rosa – sinensis*

Common names: China rose, Hawaiian hibiscus

Local name: *Igbo:* Flawa. *Yoruba:* Kekeke

History: It is native to East Asia.

Belief: It is used in the worship of Devi, and the red variety is especially prominent, having an important part in tantra

Parts used: Leaves and flowers

Local uses: The slimy liquid from leaves washed in water is used to relieve stomach upset. The flowers are purgative and are used to control menstruation. For mouth sore; leaves are washed clean, cut into pieces and add 10ml boiling water for 15 minutes filter when cold and take 3 times daily. Antiaging, anticancer, antimicrobial, diabetes, hair care, hair growth (Priya, 2014).

Chemical constituents: Gycosides, alkaloids, tannins, flavonoids, saponin and carbohydrates (Udita *et al.,* 2015).

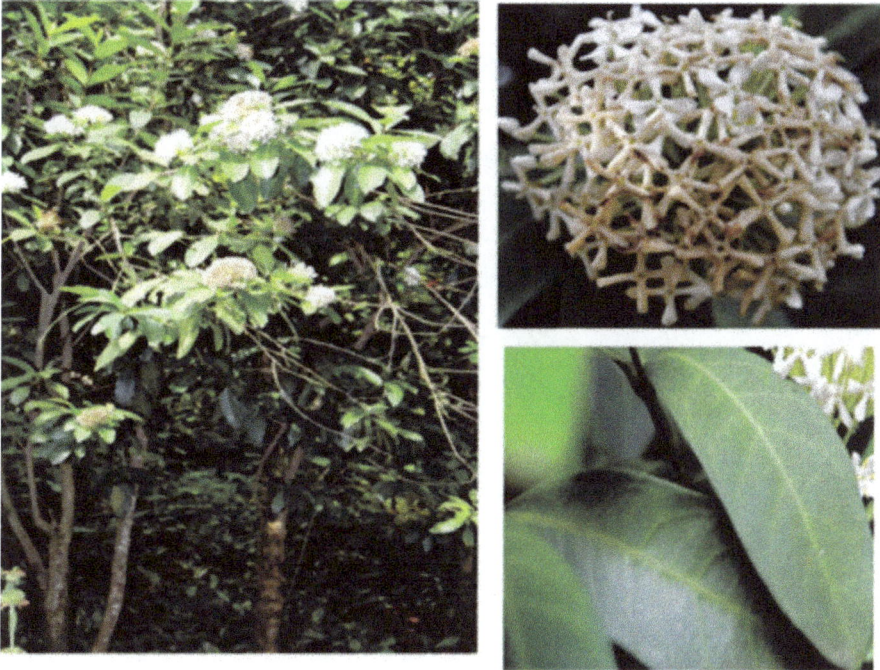

Family: Rubiaceae

Botanical name: *Ixora fillansonina*

Common name: Siamese white ixora, Fragrant ixora

History: Ixora is a genus of flowering plants in the Rubiaceae family. It is the only genus in the tribe Ixoreae. It consists of tropical evergreen trees and shrubs and holds around 545 species. Though native to the tropical and subtropical areas throughout the world, its centre of diversity is in Tropical Asia. Members of Ixora prefer acidic soil and are suitable choices for bonsai. It is also a popular choice for hedges in parts of South East Asia.

Belief: It is commonly used in Hindu worship, as well as in ayurveda and Indian folk medicine.

Local uses: Decoction of roots used for nausea, hiccups, and anorexia.

Chemical constituents: Root contains an aromatic acrid oil, tannin, fatty acids. Leaves yield flavonols; Kaemferol and quercetin, proanthocyanidins and phenolic acids and ferulic acids. Flowers contain cyanidin and Flaconboids, and a coloring material related to Quercitin.

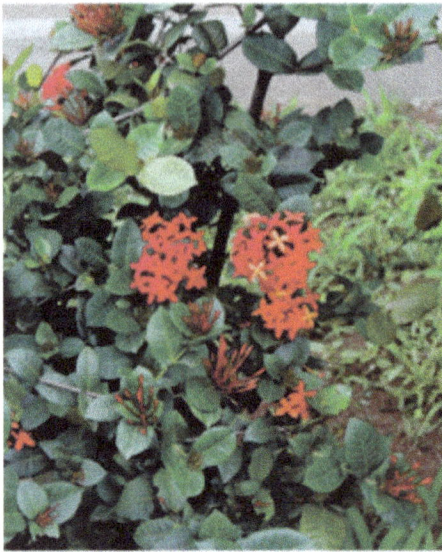

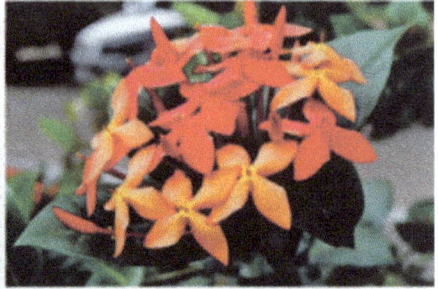

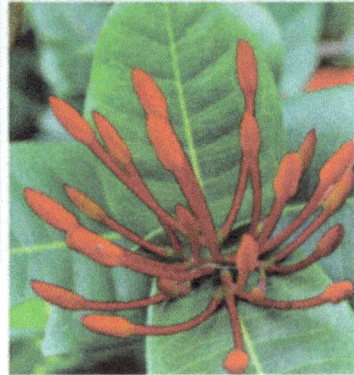

Family: Rubiaceae

Botanical name: *Ixora coccinea*

Common names: Flame of the woods, jungle flame, Jungle geranium

History: *Ixora coccinea* (also known as jungle geranium, flame of the woods or jungle flame) is a species of flowering plant in the Rubiaceae family. It is a common flowering shrub native to Southern India and Sri Lanka. It has become one of the most popular flowering shrubs in South Florida gardens and landscapes. It is the National flower of Suriname respectively.

Belief: The flowers, leaves, roots, and the stem are believed to treat various ailments in the Indian traditional system of medicine, the Ayurveda, and in various folk medicines.

Parts used: Roots, stems, leaves, flowers.

Local uses: Flowers are used for dysentery, leucorrhea. Poultice of fresh leaves and stems for sprains, eczema, boils and contusions. Decoction of the leaves is used for typhoid. Effective for treating Bronchitis and Eczema.

Chemical constituents: aromatic acrid oil, tannin, fatty acids, leaves – flavonoids, Kaemferol and quercetin, Proanthocyanidins, phenolic acids, ferulic acids.

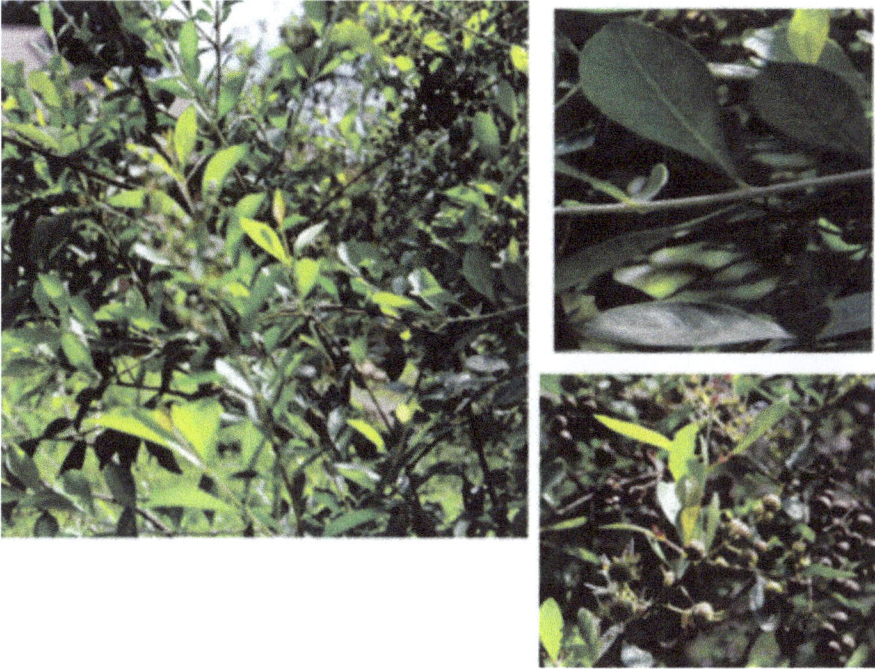

Location: Ewu

Family: Lythraceae

Botanical name: *Lawsonia inermis*

Common name: Henna, Cypress shrub, Egyptian privet

Local Name: *Edo:* Lalli. *Hausa:* Gwarzo, Lalle, Marandaa. *Yoruba:* Lalli.

History: The English name "henna" comes from the Arabic hinnā; loosely pronounced as /ħinna/. The name henna also refers to the dye prepared from the plant and the temporary body art (staining) based on those dyes. Henna has been used since antiquity to dye skin, hair and fingernails, as well as fabrics including silk, wool and leather. Historically, henna was used in the Arabian Peninsula, Indian Subcontinent, parts of South East Asia, Carthage, other parts of North Africa and the Horn of Africa. The name is used in other skin and hair dyes, such as black henna and neutral henna, neither of which is derived from the henna plant.

Belief: Some also believe that steaming or warming the henna pattern will darken the stain, either during the time the paste is still on the skin, or after the paste has been removed. It is debatable whether this adds to the color of the end result as well. After the stain reaches its peak color, it holds for a few days, then gradually wears off by way of exfoliation.

Local uses: Used in Cote d'Ivoire as an ingredient in arrow poison. Bark scales are sometimes used as a fish poison. A decoction of the bark is used as an emmenagogue, and also to treat liver problems and nervous symptoms (Uphof, 1959 and Chevallier, 1996).

Chemical constituents: Coumarins, naphthaquinones (including lawsone), flavonoids, sterols and tannins (Chevallier, 1996).

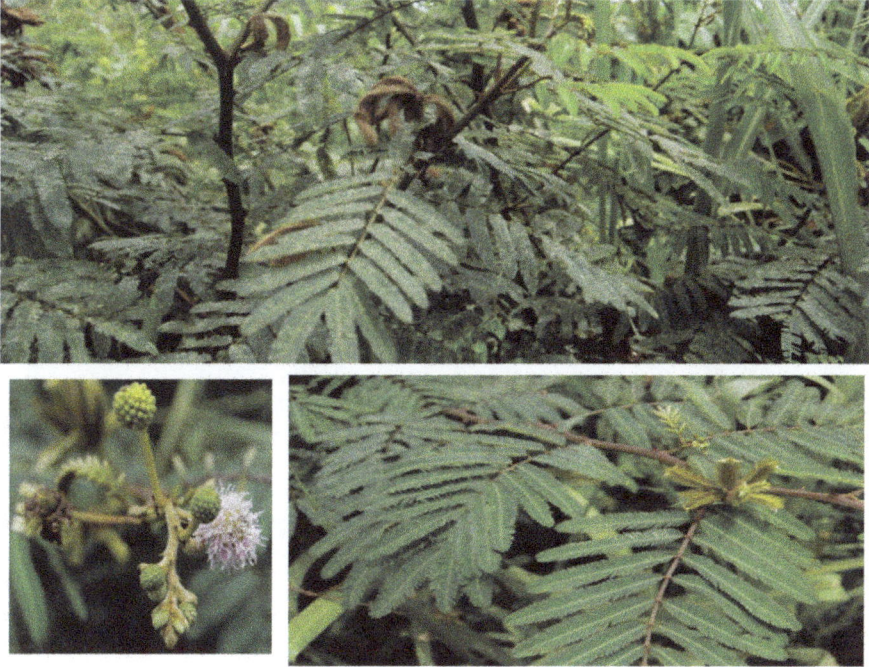

Family: Fabaceae

Botanical name: *Mimosa Pigra*

Common name: Bashful palm, Catclaw mimosa, giant seat, giant sensitive plant, thorny.

Local names: *Hausa:* Gwambe, Gumbii, kwriyaa, kaidaji, dan kunya.
Yoruba: Ewon, agogo

History: It is native to the Neotropics, but has been listed as one of the world's 100 worst invasive species and forms dense, thorny, impenetrable thickets, particularly in wet areas. The genus Mimosa (Mimosaceae) contains 400-450 species, which are mostly native to South America. *Mimosa pigra* is a woody invasive shrub that originates from tropical America and has now become widespread throughout the tropics.

Local use: The plant is used in tropical Africa as a tonic and a treatment for diarrhoea, gonorrhoea and blood poisoning. The leaf is said to contain mimosine; it is purgative and perhaps tonic. A decoction of the leaves and stems is used to treat thrush in babies and bed-wetting in children. The powdered leaf is taken with water to relieve swelling, it is used in the treatment of asthma, diarrhoea, typhoid fever and genitourinary tract infections (Sonibare and Gbile 2008).

Chemical constituents: Saponin, flavonol, glycoside (Mbatchou *et al.*, 1992).

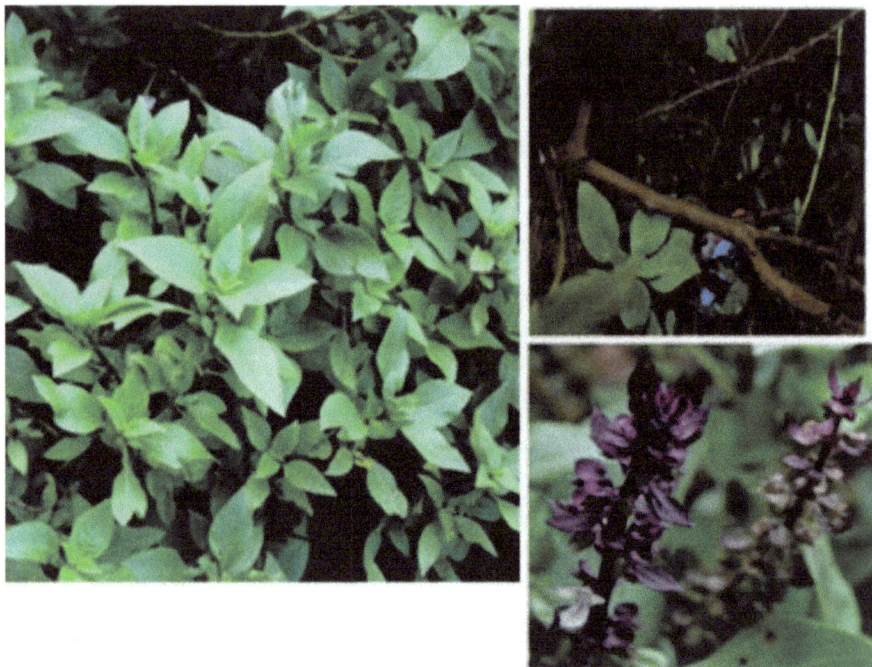

Family: Lamiaceae

Botanical name: *Ocimum kilimandscaricum*

Local uses: It is useful in cough, bronchitis, catarrh, foul ulcers and wounds, anorexia and vitiated conditions of vata and for glaucoma (Warrier et al., 1995 and Khare, 2007).

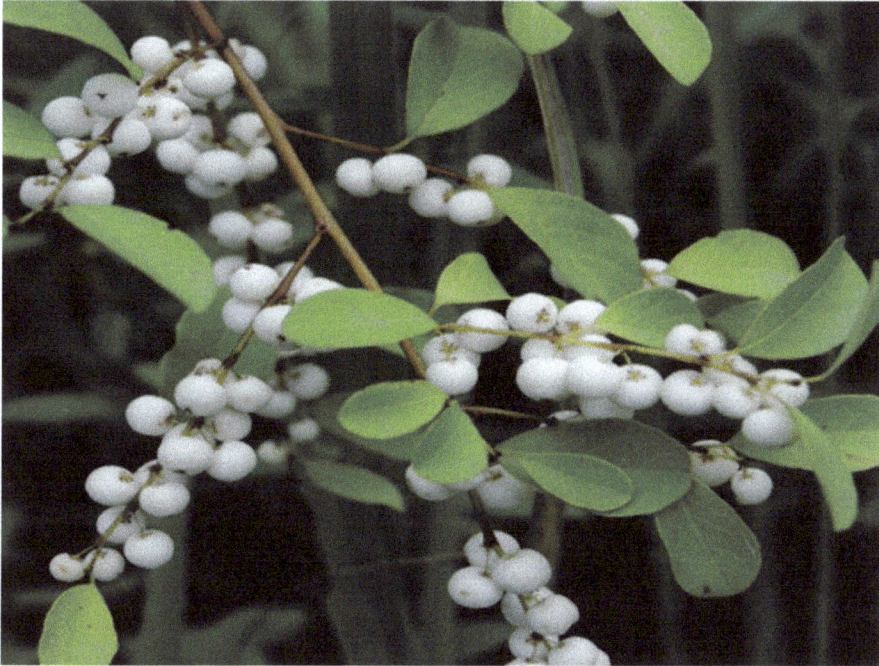

Family: Euphorbiaeceae

Botanical name: *Securinega virosa*

Common names: Whiteberry bush, snowberry tree

History: It is widely distributed throughout tropical Africa, India, Malaya, China and Australia. In Nigeria, it is found in virtually all parts of the country and in many parts of Africa including the north Eastern Nigeria.

Parts used: Root, leaves, and bark

Local uses: The leaves are used as laxatives. Root juice mixed in fat is used as a soothing ointment. Bark is an astringent for diarrhoea and dysentery. It is an analgesic and it is also used for abscesses and anaemia.

Chemical constituents: Alkaloids (Securine), tannins and carbohydrates.

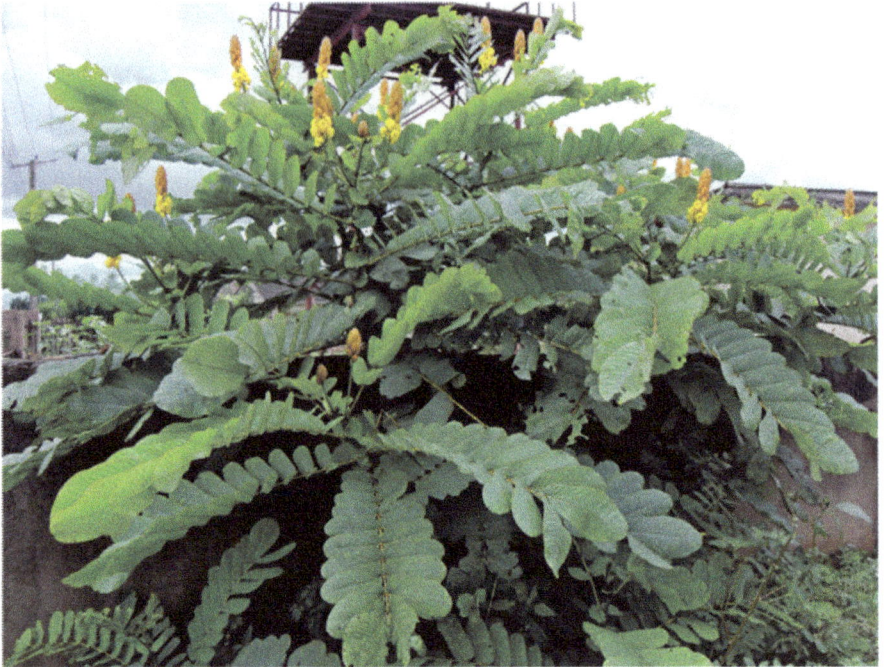

Family: Caesalpinaceae

Botanical name: *Senna alata*

Common names: Senna, ring worm plant

Local name: *Igbo:* Ogalu, Ndiuchi. *Yoruba:* Asunrun Oyinbo

History: It is native to Mexico, and can be found in diverse habitats.

Parts used: Whole plant

Local Uses: The entire plant is used for the treatment of venereal diseases in women. Infusion or decoction of the leaf is used as a mild laxative and a purgative in large doses. For treating ringworm and other fungal infections of the skin. The leaves are ground in a mortar to obtain a kind of green cotton wool. This is mixed with the same amount of vegetable oil and rubbed on the affected area two or three times a day. A fresh preparation is made every day (Hirt, *et al.,* 2008).

Chemical constituents: Anthraquninoes, szulene, saponin

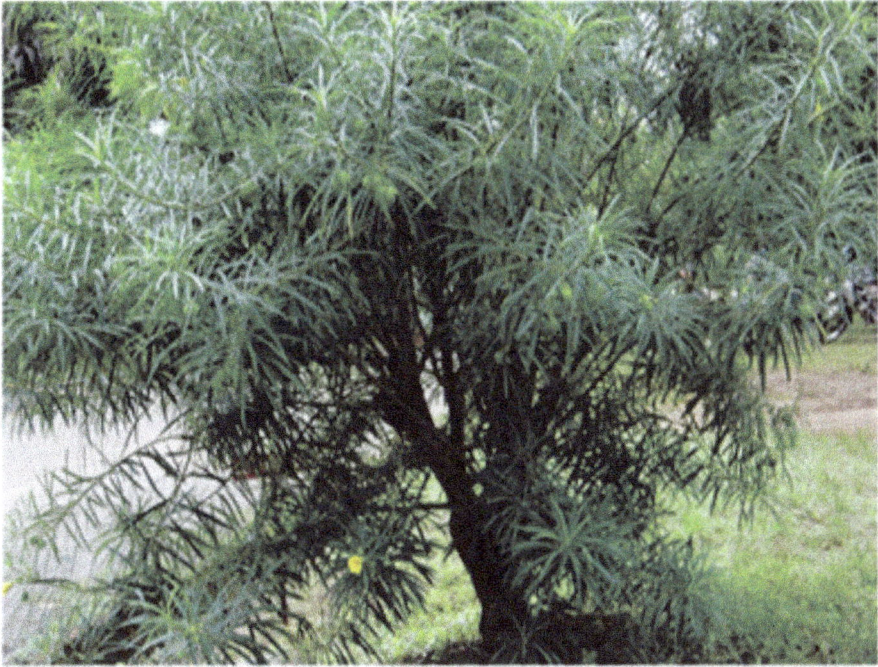

Family: Apocynaceae

Botanical name: *Thevetia nerifolia*

Common names: Exile tree, yellow oleander

History: A shrub to 6 m high, native of central and tropical S America from Mexico and the West Indies to Brazil.

Belief: It is believed that the plant's toxicity is comparable to the venom of a rattlesnake.

Parts used: Leaves, stem, bark, kernel

Local Uses: All parts of these plants are toxic (especially the seeds) and contain a variety of cardiac glycosides including thevetins A and B. Ingestion of yellow oleander results in nausea, vomiting, abdominal pain, diarrhoea, cardiac dysrhythmias, and hyperkalemia (Bandara et al., 2010 and Roberts et al., 2006).

Chemical constituents: Nerifolin, Cardenolides-thevetin a & b (Bandara et al., 2010).

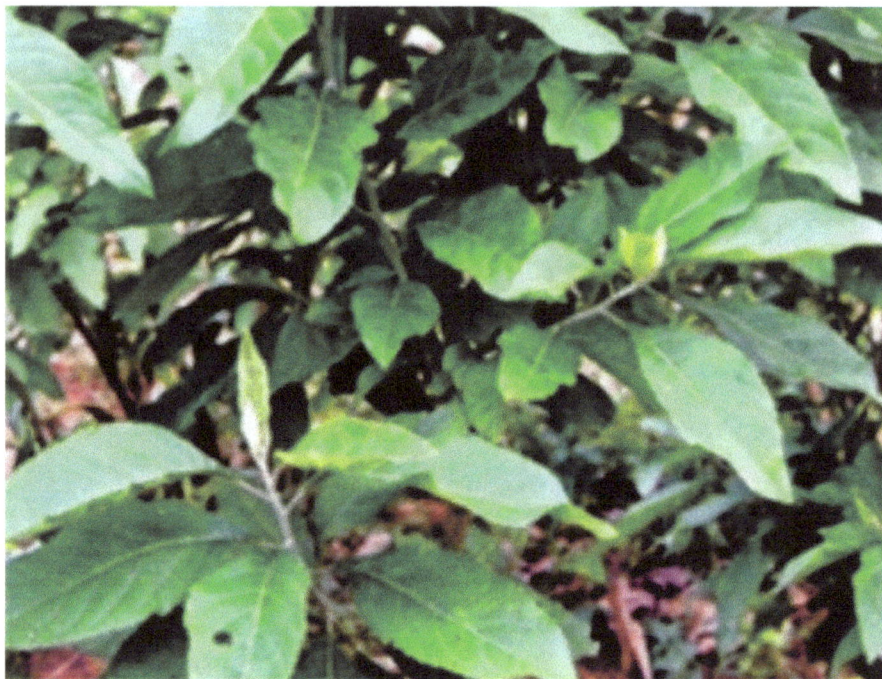

Family: Asteraceae

Botanical name: *Vernonia amygdalina*

Common names: Bitter leaf

History: A member of the Asteraceae family, it is a small shrub that grows in tropical Africa.

Belief: It is consumed by Hausa female of the Northern Nigeria with the belief that it enhances sexual attraction.

Parts used: Bark, root, leaves and fruits.

Local uses: In a preliminary clinical trial, a decoction of 25 g fresh leaves of *V. amygdalina* was 67% effective in creating an adequate clinical response in African patients with mild falciparum malaria (Challand and Willcox, 2009). Enhances the immune system. Many studies have shown that V. amygdalina extracts may strengthen the immune system through many cytokines (including NFKB, pro inflammatory molecule) regulation (Sweeney *et al.,* 2005).

Chemical constituents: sesquiterpene lactones (Vernodalin, Vernolepin and Vernomygdin) and Steroid Glucosides (Calixto, 2000; Smith, 2008 and Finar, 2008)

References

Akindele, A. J. and Adeyemi O. O. (2007). Antiinflammatory activity of the aqueous leaf extract of Byrsocarpus coccineus Fitoterapia, 78: 25-28.

Akindele, A. J., Ezenwanebe, K. O., Anunobi, C.C. and Adeyemi, O. O. (2010). Hepatoprotective and in vivo antioxidant effectsof Byrsocarpus coccineus Schum. and Thonn. (Connaraceae.). J Ethnopharmacol,129: 46-52.

Ambasta, S. P. (2004). The useful plants of India. National Institute of Science Communication. New Delhi, 4th ed. pp. 94–5.11.

Bandara, A., Scott, A. Weinstein, J. W. and Michael, E. (2010). A review of the natural history, toxicology, diagnosis and clinical management of Nerium oleander and Thevetia peruviana

Bressani, R., Gómez-Brenes, R. A., Elías, L. G. H. (1986). "Nutritional quality of pigeon pea protein, immature and ripe, and its supplementary value for cereals". Arch Latinoam Nutr.,36 (1): 108–16.

Brunner JH. 1984. Direct Spectrophotometric determination of Saponins. Anal. Chem., 34:1314-1326.

Calixto J.B. (2000): Efficacy, safety, and quality control, marketing egulatory guidelines for herbals (phytotherapeutic agents). Braz. J. Med. Biol. Res., 33:179 – 189.

Challand, S., Willcox, M. (2009). A clinical trial of the traditional medicine Vernonia amygdalina in the treatment of uncomplicated malaria. J. Altern. Complement Med., 15 (11): 1231–7.

Chevallier. A (1996). The Encyclopedia of Medicinal Plants Publication. London: Dorling Kindersley Publishers.

DeFilipps, R. A.; Maina, S. L.; & Crepin, J. Medicinal Plants of the\ Guianas. http://botany.si.edu/bdg/medicinal/index.html. Smithsonian Museum Publisher

Dosseh K, Kpatcha T, Adjrah Y, Idoh K, Agbonon A, Gbéassor M 2014). Anti-inflammatory effect of Byrsocarpus coccineus chum. and Thonn. (Connaraceae) root. World J. Pharm. Res. 3:3585-3598.

el-Deeb KS (2003). The volatile constituents in the absolute of Clerodendron splendens G Don flower oil. Bull Fac Pharm Cairo Univ.41:259–63.

Ettebong E, and Nwafor P (2009). In vitro antimicrobial activities of extracts of carpolobia lutea root. Pak J Pharm Sci. 22(3):335–338.

Finar I.L., (2008): Organic chemistry vol. 2; Stereochemistry and the chemistry of natural products. 5th Edition. Saurabh printers Pvt Ltd. India. Pp 956

Fitoterapia, 71: 77–79.

Gupta M, Mazumdhar UK, Gomathi P (2007). Evaluation of antipyretic and antinociceptive activities of Plumeria acuminata leaves. J Med Sci. 7: 835-839.

Hirt, H. M. and Bindanda M. (2008). Natural Medicine in the Tropics I: Foundation text. anamed, Winnenden, Germany

Igboko, D. O. 1983. Phytochemical studies on Garcinia Kola Heckel. M. Sc Thesis. University of Nigeria, Nsukka. 202.

Irvine, F. R (1961). Woody plants of Ghana. 1st ed. UK: Oxford University Press; p.74.

Khare, C.P. (2007) Indian Medicinal plants: An illustrated Dictionary. pringer Science? Business Media, Spring Street, New York, p 445

Kumar, V. L. and Basu, N. (1994). Anti-inflammatory activity of the latex of Calotropis procera, J. Ethanopharmacol. 44, 123–5

Mainasara, M. M., Aliero B. L., Aliero A. A., and Dahiru S. S. (2011 Phytochemical and Antibacterial Properties of Calotropis Procera (Ait) R. Br. (Sodom Apple) Fruit and Bark Extracts, International Journal of Modern Botany, Vol. 1 No. 1, 2011, pp. 8-11.

Mbatchou V.C., Ayebila A.J. and Apea O.B. (1992). Antibacterial activity of phytochemicals from Acacia nilotica, Entada africana and Mimosa pigra L. on Salmonela typhi. J. Anim. Plant Sci., 10 (1) 1248-1258

Merina AJ, Sivanesan D, Hazeena V and Sulochana N (2010 Antioxidant and hypolipidemic effect of Plumeria rubra L. in alloxan induced hyperglycemic rats. E-Journal of Chemistry, 7: 1-5.

Mikhail O.A and Musbau Adewumi, 2013. Phytochemical and mineral constituents of Cochlospermum planchonii (Hook. Ef. x Planch) Root. Bioresearch Bulletin

Ocimum kilimandscharicum Guerke (Lamiaceae): A New Distributional Record for Peninsular India with Focus on its Economic Potential (PDF Download Available). Available from: https://www.researchgate.net/publication/ 276096752_Ocimum_ kilimandscharicum_

Guerke_Lamiaceae_A_New_ Distributional_Record_for_Peninsular_India_with_Focus_on_ its_Economic_Potential [accessed Oct 27 2017].

Pauline D.P. (2000). Plants Used In Cambodia, printed by Imprimerie Olympic, Phnom Penh poisoning, Toxicon official journal of the International Society on Toxicology, Volume 56(3, 1): 273-281 Priya Nair (2014). Health benefits of Hibiscus rosa sinensis. Value Food: Nutrition and Health Information Portal, http:// www.value-food.info

Protabase-Plant Resources of Tropical Africa. http://www.prota.org Roberts D.M, Southcott E and Potter J.M, Roberts, Buckley N.A. (2006): "Pharmacokinetics of digoxin cross-reacting substances in patients with acute yellow oleander (Thevetia peruviana) poisoning, including the effect of activated charcoal." Therapeutic Drug Monitoring, 28:6 (784-792)

Salah W, Miller N, Pagauga G, Tybury G, Bolwell E, Rice E, and Evans C. (1995). Polyphenolic flavonoids as scavenger of aqueous phase radicals and chain breaking antioxidants. Arch. Biochem. 2:239-46.

Sharma P and Sharma JD (2000). In vitro Schizonticidal screening of Calotropis procera

Shehata AH, Yousif MF, Soliman GA (2001). Phytochemical and Pharmacological investigation of Clerodendron splendens G. Don growing in Egypt. Egypt J Biomed Sci.7:145–63.

Singh Baghel A. (2010). Antibacterial activity of Plumeria rubra Linn. Plant Extract., Journal of Chem. Pharm. Res., 2(6):435-440

Smith G.J., (2008): Organic chemistry.2nd Edition. McGraw-Hill publishers. New York. Pp 1175

Sonibare M.A., and Gbile Z.O. (2008). Ethnobotanical survey of anti-asthmatic plants in South Western Nigeria. Afr. J. Compliment. Altern. Med., 5 (4) 340-345

Sweeney CJ, Mehrotra S, Sadaria MR, Kumar S, Shortle NH, Roman Y, Sheridan C, Campbell RA, Murray DJ, Badve S, Nakshatri H (2005). "The sesquiterpene lactone parthenolide in combination with docetaxel reduces metastasis and improves survival in a xenograft model of breast cancer". Mole. Cancer Ther. 4 (6): 1004.

Udita T., Poonam Y. and Darshika N. (2015). Study on Phytochemical Screening and Antibacterial Potential of Methanolic Flower and Leaf Extracts of Hibiscus rosa sinensis. International Journal of Innovative and Applied Research, 3(6): 9- 14

Uphof. J. C. Th. (1959). Dictionary of Economic Plants. Weinheim Publisher.

Warrier PK, Nambiar VPK and Ramankutty C (1995) In: Varier PS (ed) Indian medicinal plants: a compendium of 500 species, 4. 157–168 Rep (2003)

Yakubu MT, Akanji MA and Nafiu MO. (2010). Anti-diabetic activity of aqueous extract of Cochlospermum planchonii root in alloxan- induced diabetic rats. Cameroon J. Expt Biol, 6(2):91-100.

Yuan-gang Zu, Xiao-lei ,Yu-jie Fu, Nan Wu, YuKong, Michael W (2010). Chemical composition of the SFE-CO2 extracts from Cajanus cajan (L.) Huth and their antimicrobial activity in vitro and in vivo. Phytomed, 17:1095–101.

Chapter 5

Forbs

A forb (sometimes spelled phorb) is a herbaceous flowering plant that is not a graminoid (grasses, sedges and rushes). The term is used in biology and in vegetation ecology, especially in relation to grasslands. This chapter takes an exciting forage into the world of forbs, how they are used by traditional healers in treating diseases, the local taboos surrounding these plants and the scientific basis, if any, of the uses.

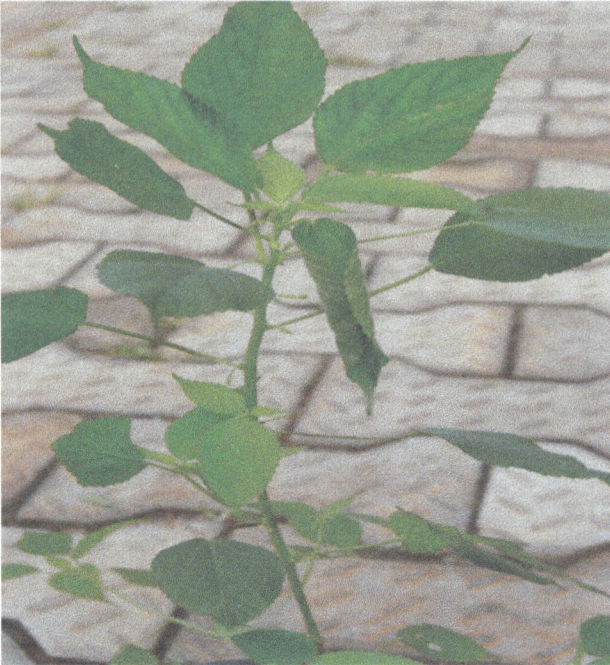

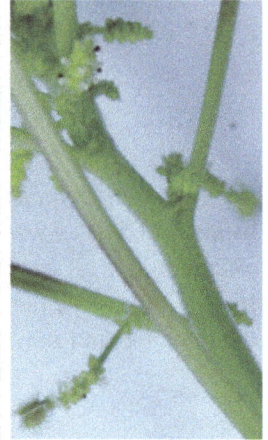

Family: Euphorbiaceae

Botanical name: *Acalypha ciliata*

Common name: Copper leaf plant

Local name: *Esan:* Ifoki. *Igbo:* Abaleba *Yoruba:* Ẹfiri

History: It occurs widely in Africa where it is eaten as a vegetable, or fed to animals. In West Africa and East Africa, it is used as a medicinal plant.

Local uses: Leaves - cooked and eaten as a vegetable, it is said to be eaten with okra *(Abelmoschatus esculentus)* or the leaves of *Vigna unguiculata.* A decoction of the leaves is drunk as a remedy for female sterility, the mashed leaves are applied as a dressing to sores. It occurs widely in Africa where it is eaten as a vegetable or fed to animals (Goode, 1989). In West Africa and East Africa it is used as a medicinal plant (Schmelzer and Gurib-Fakim, 2008).

Chemical constituents: Alkaloid, flavonoid, saponin, tanin (Odeja, 2007).

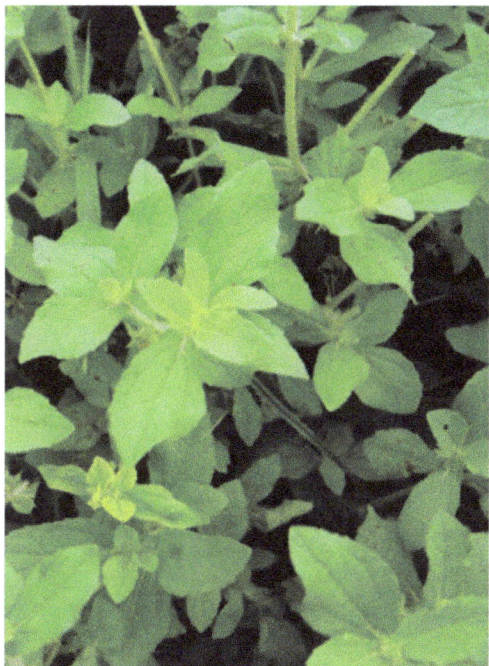
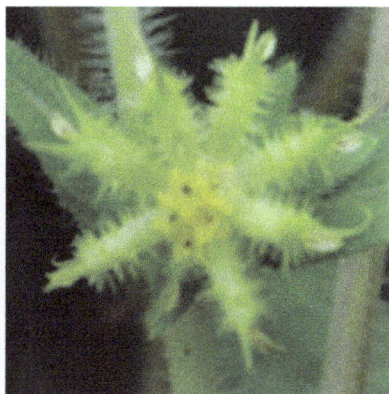

Family: Asteraceae

Botanical name: *Acanthospermum hispidum*

Common name: Bristly starbur, Goat's head, Hispid starbur, Starbur

History: It is an annual plant in the family Asteraceae, which is native to Central and South America. It is also naturalized in many scattered places in Eurasia, Africa, North America.

Local uses: In India, the seeds are ingested orally to treat bed wetting, while in Malaysia, the entire plant is mixed with castor oil and applied to the skin to treat scabies. Corrêa (1926) compiled a basic compendium of medicinal plants in Brazil, and described the use from the roots of *A. hispidum* to treat coughs and bronchitis, while noting that the seeds are toxic to Chickens,

Chemical constituents: alkaloid, tannin, flavonoid, saponin, glycoside

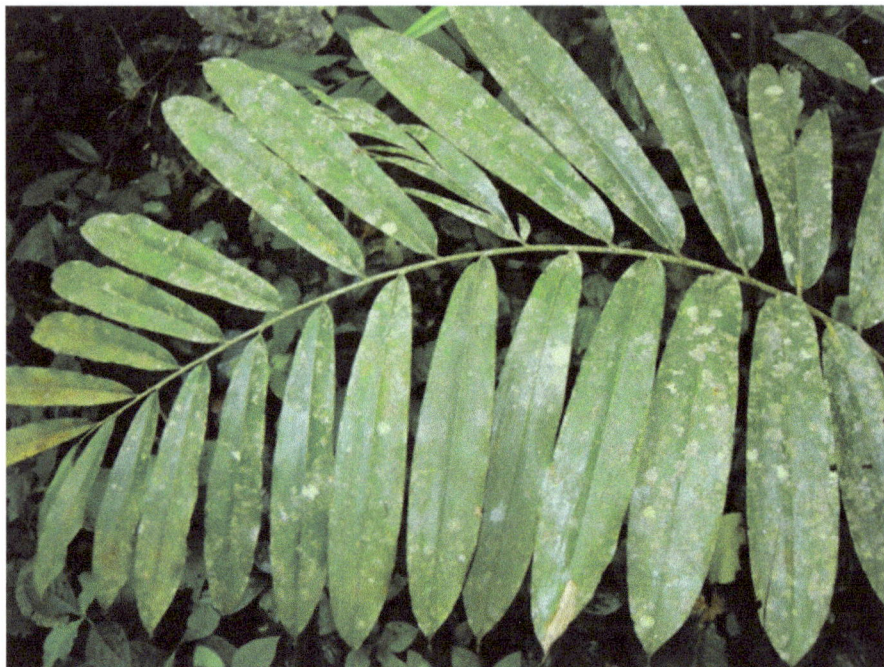

Family: Zingiberaceae

Botanical name: *Aframomum alboviolaceum*

Common name: Broad amomum, Aframomum africanum fruit or grape-seeded amomum

History: *Aframomum alboviolaceum* is a species of dicotyledonous plants of the family Zingiberaceae, originating in tropical Africa

Local use: Its leaves are used as spice and its seeds for stomachic purposes and vermifuge.

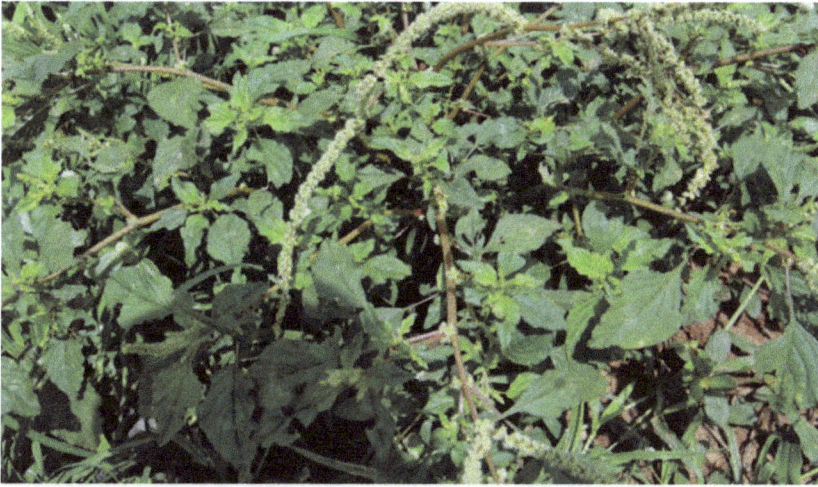

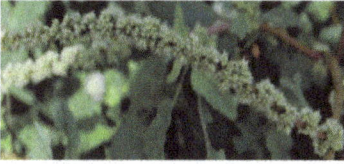

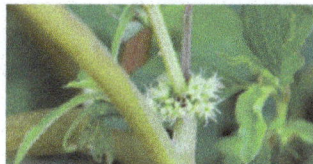

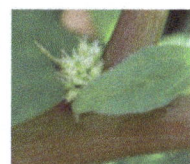

Family: Asteraceae

Botanical name: *Ageratum conyzoides*

Common names: Billy goat weed

Local names: *Edo:* Ebi-ighedore. *Igbo:* Oranjila. *Yoruba:* Imi-esu

History: Ageratum is derived from the Greek "a geras," meaning nonaging, referring to the longevity of the flowers or the whole plant. The specific epithet "conyzoides" is derived from "kónyz," the Greek name of Inula helenium, which it resembles (Kissmann and Groth, 1993).

Belief: The plant is believed to have a rank smell, likened in Australia to that of a male goat, hence the common name billy goat weed.

Local uses: It is used to treat wounds and burns. A decotion of the plant is used as a lotion for scabies (craw-craw) and drunk as a remedy for fever. The juice of the leaves is dropped in the eyes to cure inflammations. As a medicinal plant, *Ageratum conyzoides* is widely used by many traditional cultures, especially as an antidysenteric. It is also an insecticide and nematicide (Ming, 1999).

Chemical constituents: Flavonoids, alkaloids, cumarins, essential oils, and tannins (Jaccoud, 1961).

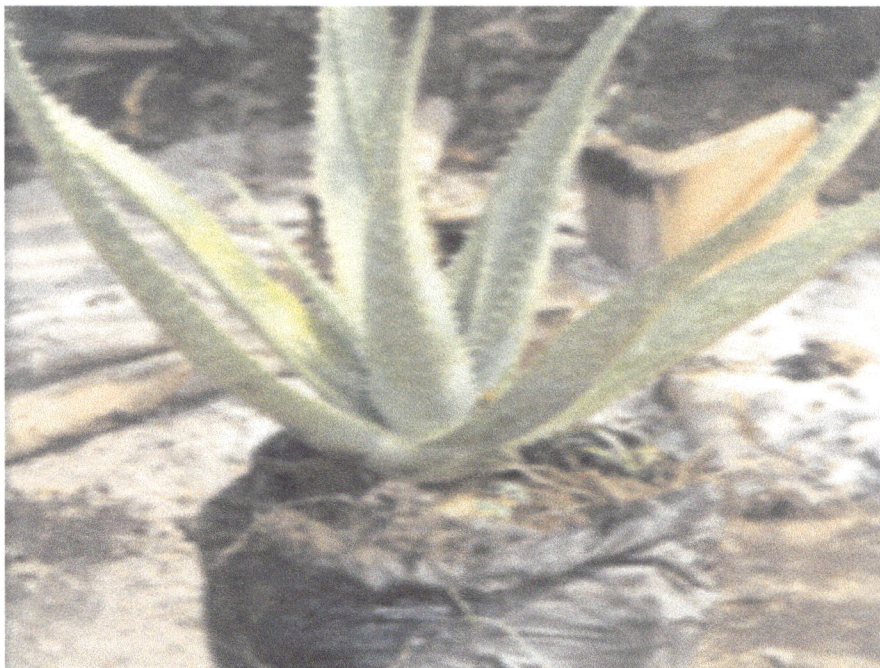

Family: Liliaceae

Botanical name: *Aloe barteri*

Common names: Aloevera

History: From the Mediterranean region, it was carried to the New World in the 16th century by Spanish explorers and missionaries. In the modern era, its clinical use began in the 1930s as a treatment for *roentgen dermatitis* (Grindlay and Reynolds, 1986).

Belief: The leaves of *Aloe barteri* (syn *Aloe buettneri*) can be applied externally and is believed to help skin conditions such as burns, wounds, insect bites, Guinea worm sores and vitiligo.

Local uses: It is used for the treatment of typhoid fever. It is used to treat skin wounds, burn, scald, blisters, insects bite, applied externally, it is believed to help skin conditions such as burns, wounds, insect bites, Guinea worm sores and vitiligo (Burkill, 1995).

Chemical constituents: Aloe resin is the solid residue obtained by evaporating the latex from the pericyclic cells beneath the skin (Leung and Foster, 1980). Tannins, polysaccharides, organic acids, enzymes, vitamins, and steroids, have been identified (Henry, 1979).

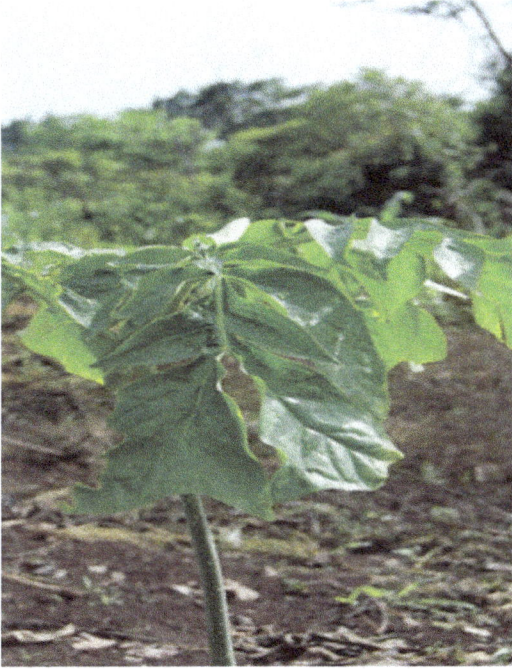

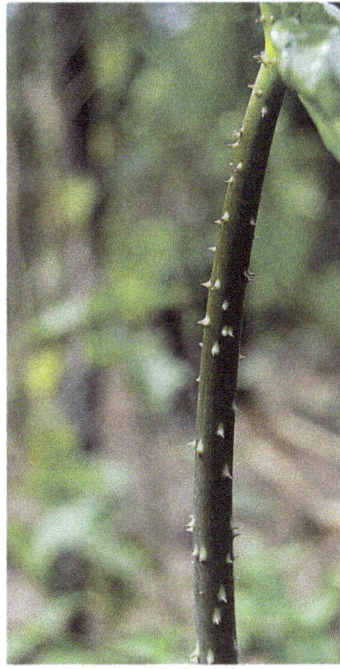

Family: Araceae

Botanical name: *Anchomanes difformis*

Common names: Aroids

Local names: *Edo:* Olikhoror. *Igbo:* Oje. *Yoruba:* Iwaja

History: It is commonly found in West Africa, occurring in the forest of Sierra Leone to W Cameroons.

Belief: Believed to sub-serve medicinal properties

Parts used: Stem and Leaves

Local uses: Leaf and tuber are used as a lactation stimulant. The plant is used locally for medicinal purposes, and the tuber is harvested from the wild as an emergency food in times of need. The root, pulped with potter's clay, is applied to maturate abscesses (Burkil, 1985). People with a tendency to rheumatism, arthritis, gout, kidney stones and hyperacidity should take especial caution if including this plant in their diet (Bown, 1995).

Chemical constituents: saponins, tannins and alkaloids (Oyetayo, 2007)

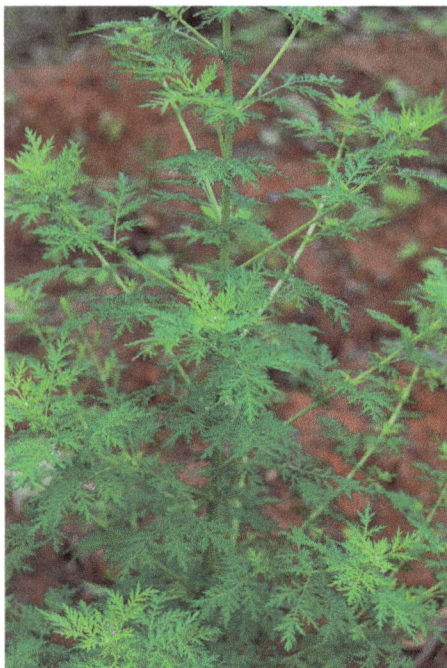

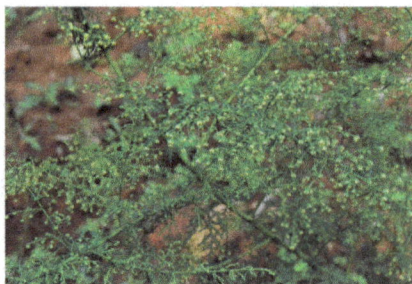

Family: Asteraceae

Botanical name: *Artemisia annua*

Common names: Annual worm wood, Sweet annie, Sweet worm wood

History: Is a common type of wormwood native to temperate Asia, but naturalized in many countries including scattered parts of North America.

Belief: Believed by local people to heal diseases and eliminates evil.

Parts used: Whole plant

Local uses: It is used in the treatment of malaria, fevers, haemorrhoids. Used in crafting of aromatic, wreaths, as flavouring for spirits such as vermouth. Sweet annie (add,) is an aromatic annual herb which is the source of artemisinin and essential oils. (Simon *et al.,* 1990). The secondary plant product artemisinin known in Chinese folk medicine as qinghasu is an antimalarial with reduced side effects compared to quinine, chloroquine or other antimalarial (Klayman, 1985).

Chemical constituents: The major active constituent of *Artemisia annua*, *Artemisia apiacea*, and *Artemisia lancea* is artemisinin. Derivatives of this compound include arteether, artemether, artemotil, artenimol, artesunate, and dihydroartemisinin, which, along with artemisin, are currently being used to treat drug-resistant and non-drug resistant malaria (Heide, 2006; Hsu, 2006; Li, and Wu, 1998; Phan, 2002 and Lommen *et al.,* 2006).

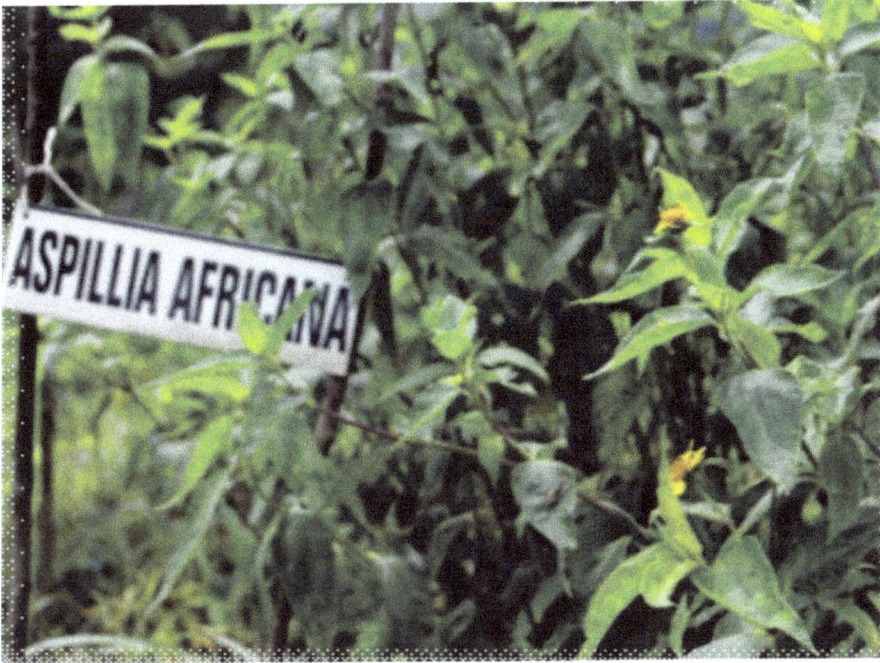

Family: Asteraceae

Botanical name: *Aspilia africana*

Common names: Haemorrhage plant, African marigold, Wild sun flower

Parts used: Leaves and roots

Local uses: Historically, *Aspilia africana* was used in Mbaise and most Igbo speaking parts of Nigeria to prevent conception, suggesting potential contraceptive and anti-fertility properties (Oluyemi, 2007). Leaf extract and fractions of *A. africana* effectively arrested bleeding from fresh wounds, inhibited microbial growth of known wound contaminants and accelerated wound healing process.

Chemical constituents: Alkaloid, Tannin, Saponin, Phylobatannin, Terpenoid Flavonoid and Cardiac glycoside (Oko and Agiang, 2001).

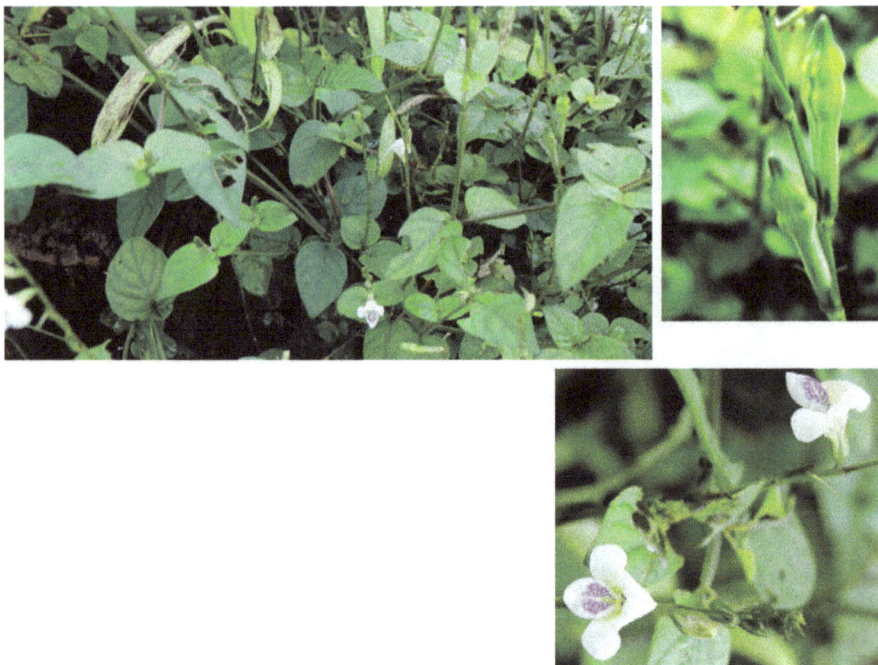

Family: Acanthaceae

Botanical name: *Asystacia gigantica*

Common name: Cripping fox glove, Chinese violet

Local name: *Edo:* Ebe ogboghiro. *Yoruba:* Oseta

History: It is a species of plant in the Acanthaceae family. It is commonly known as the Chinese violet, coromandel or creeping foxglove. In South Africa this plant may simply be called asystasia.

Local uses: In some parts of Africa, the leaves are eaten as a vegetable and used as an herbal remedy in traditional African medicine. The leaves are used in many parts of Nigeria as a traditional African medicine for the management of asthma. The plant is used in ethnomedicine for the treatment of heart pains, stomach pains, rheumatism, as vermifuge and anthelmintic (Chopra, 1933 and Kokwaro, 1976) It is also used as an ornamental plant.

Chemical constituents: Saponin, reducing sugar, Steroids, Glycosides, Flavonoids and Anthraquinones (Hamid et al., 2001).

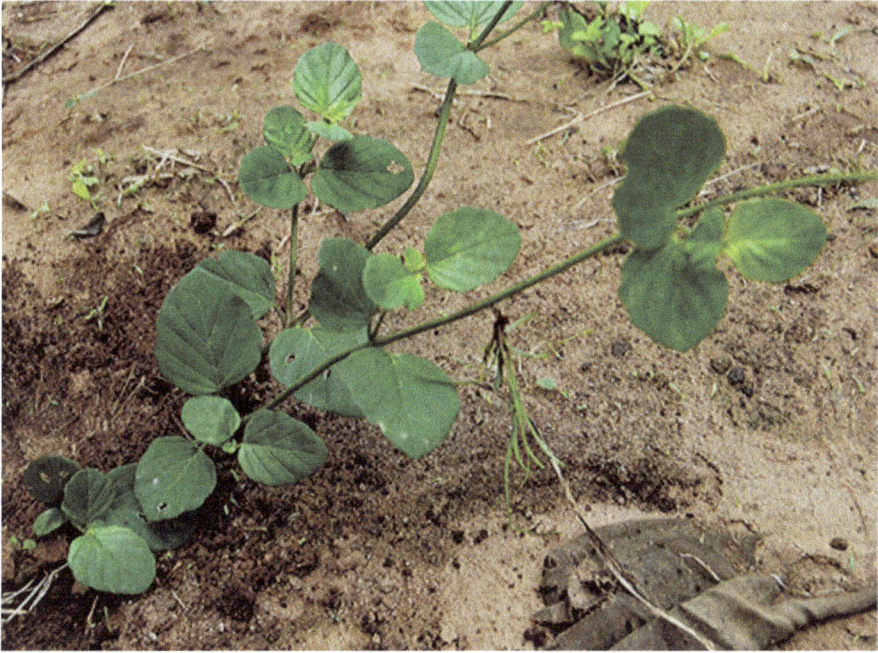

Family: Nyctaginaceae

Botanical name: *Boerhavia diffusa*

Common names: Hog weed, spiderlings

History: *Boerhavia diffusa* is a species of flowering plant in the family which is commonly known as punarnava (meaning that which rejuvenates or renews the body in Ayurveda),

Belief: *Boerhavia diffusa* is widely dispersed, occurring throughout India, the Pacific, and southern United States.

Parts used: Root, leaves and seed.

Local uses: In arthritis: it helps to reduce inflammation and pain in joints. In indigestion: it acts as a carminative, increases appetite, helps digestion and reduces abdominal pain. It also relieves constipation. In Ayurveda, It has been classified as "rasayana" herb which is said to possess properties like antiaging, re-establishing youth, strengthening life and brain power, and disease prevention, all of which imply that they increase the resistance of the body against any onslaught, in other words, providing hepatoprotection and immunomodulation (Govindarajan, 2005).

Chemical constituents: It contains various categories of secondary metabolites, Flavonoid glycosides, Isoflavonoids (rotenoids), Steroids (ecdysteroid), alkaloids, and Phenolic and Lignan glycosides. Recently a rapid method was developed for quantitative estimation of Boeravinones in the plant (Bairwa, 2014).

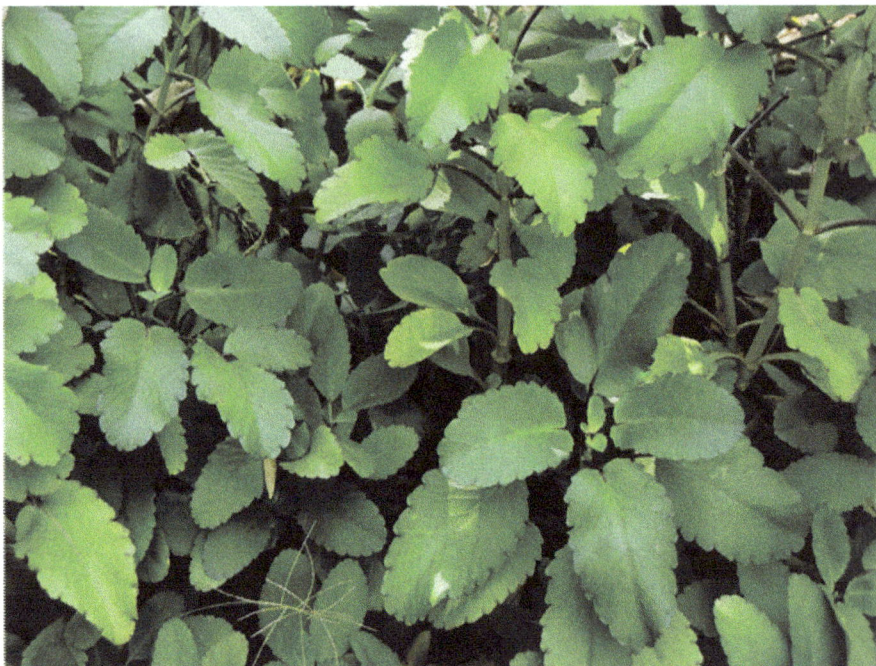

Family: Crassulaceae

Botanical name: *Bryophyllum pinnatum*

Common names: Resurrection plant, african never die, Mother of millions.

Local names: *Edo:* Okekwe. *Igbo:* Nkwonkwu, Oda opuo. *Yoruba:* Odundun

History: *Bryophyllum pinnatum,* also known as the air plant, cathedral bells, life plant, miracle leaf, and Goethe plant is a succulent plant native to Madagascar, which is a popular houseplant and has become naturalized in tropical and subtropical areas. It is distinctive for the profusion of miniature plantlets that form on the margins of its Phylloclades, a trait it has in common with some other members of its genus.

Parts used: Leaves and Roots.

Local uses: Poultice is used for treating intestinal pains. It is used as diuretic and antihelminthic. Leaves are chewed with some slices of onions for high blood pressure and stroke. Similarly, for convulsion and epilepsy (leaves with some slices of onions and plantain roots). Pounded leaf is applied to soothe inflammation. Bryophyllum pinnatum has been recorded in Trinidad and Tobago as being used as a traditional treatment for hypertension (Lans, 2006).

Chemical constituents: Bufadienolide bryophillin A which showed strong anti-tumor promoting activity in vitro, and bersaldegenin-3- acetate and bryophillin C which were less active. Bryophillin C also showed insecticidal properties (Supratman et al., 2001 and Supratman et al., 2000).

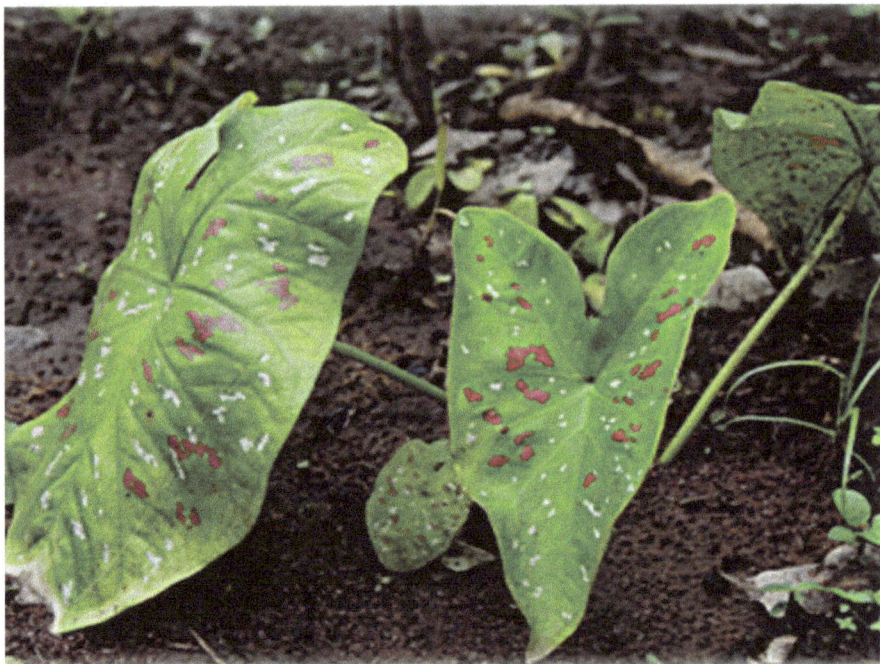

Family: Araceae

Botanical name: *Caladium bicolor*

Common names: Wild cocoyam

Local names: *Igbo*: Ede-ohia, Ede-mmuo. *Yoruba:* Eje-jesu, Lefunlosun
History: The genus Caladium includes seven species that are native to South America and Central America, and naturalized in India, parts of Africa, and various tropical islands.

Parts used: Leaves, Bulb

Local uses: Extract of fresh leaves are applied to the eyes to cure convulsion. It is also applied on the body for skin discolouration. Facial paralysis is treated by crushing the bulbs of the plants and applying to the face. Powdered tuber employed to treat facial skin blemishes by the French Guiana Palikur. All parts of the leaf are macerated in fresh water for an external bath to remedy numerous maladies of French Guiana Wayapi children. Crushed leaves are used in veterinary medicine to destroy vermin on sores of cattle. (Grenand, *et al.,* 1987; Duke, 1985 and May, 1982).

Chemicalconstituents: Alkaloids, tannins, saponin and cardiac glycoside. (Emmanuel, 2015).

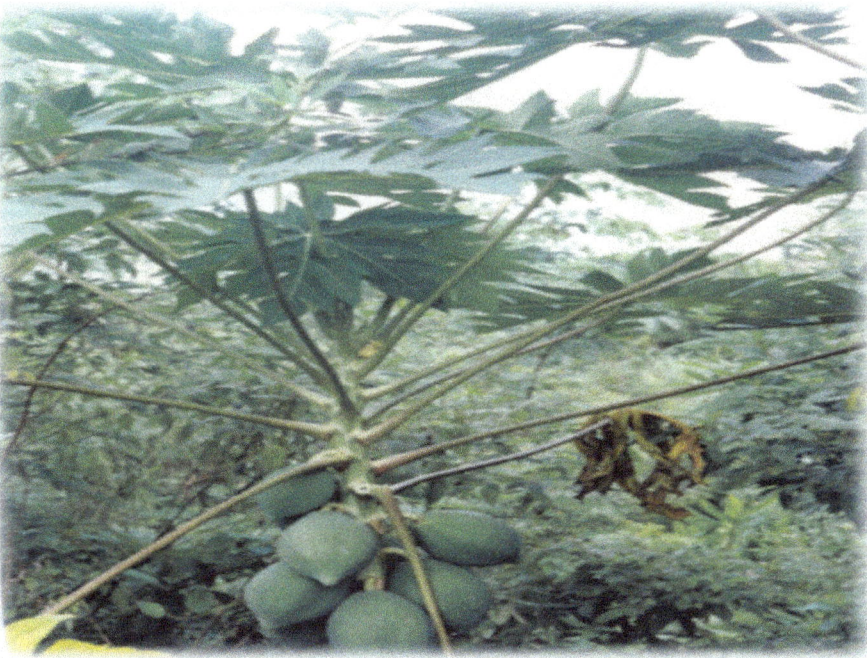

Family: Caricaceae

Botanical name: *Carica papaya*

Common names: Pawpaw

Local names: *Edo:* Uhoro. *Igbo:* Okwuru bekee. *Hausa:* Gwandar masar. *Yoruba:* Ibepe

History: Its origin is in the tropics of the Americas, perhaps from southern Mexico and neighboring Central America

Parts used: Leaves, Latex, Roots, Fruits and Seeds.

Local uses: Fruits is applied on ring worm, Leaves are taken for malaria. Leaves mixed with lemon grass and guava leaves are used in the treatment of hypertension. Source of papain, a tenderizer. Leaves are cooked with other plants to reduce fever. In some parts of the world, papaya leaves are made into tea as a treatment for malaria, but the mechanism is not understood and no treatment method based on these results has been scientifically proven (Titanji, 2008).

Chemical constituents: carotenoids and polyphenols as well as benzyl isothiocyanates and benzyl glucosinates, with skin and pulp levels that increase during ripening. Papaya seeds also contain the cyanogenic substance prunasin (Rivera-Pastrana et al., 2010; Rossetto *et al.,* 2008 and Seigler *et al.,* 2002)

115

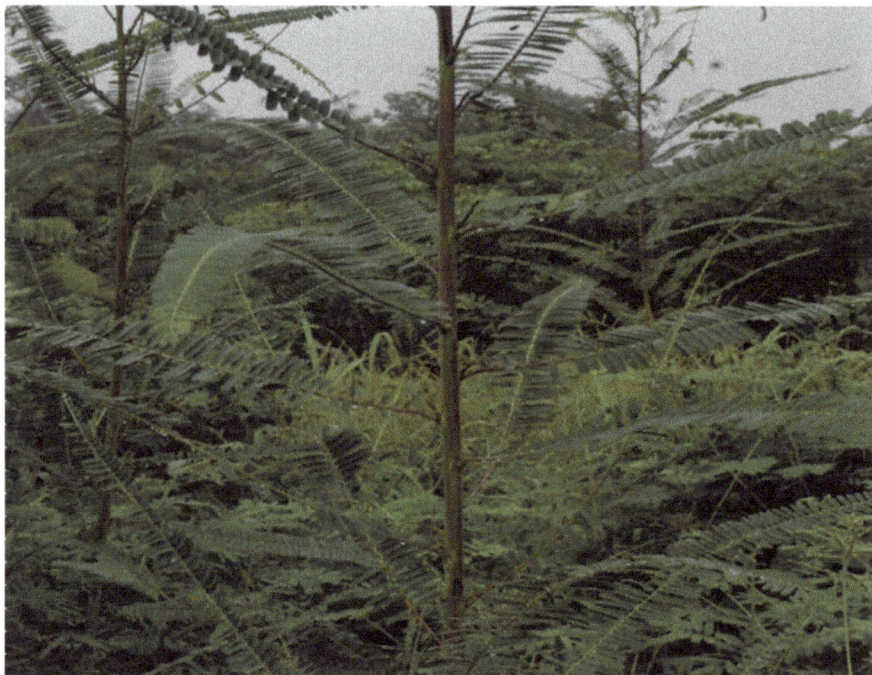

Family: Fabaceae

Botanical name: *Chamaecrista mimosoides*

Local uses: In Japan, young stems and leaves are dried and used as a substitute for tea. An aqueous extract from leaves, stems and pods called "hamacha" is a conventional beverage in the San-in district of Japan. In Japan, raw material used as diuretic or antidote in folk remedy (Hemen and Lalita, 2012).

Chemical constituents: Anthraquinones reported from seeds (physcion, physcion-9-antrhone, emodine-9-anthrone, and physcion 10, 10-bianthrone; aerial parts (chrysophanol, physcion, and emodin). Ethanol extract yielded eight compounds: Emodin, luteolin, 1,3-benzenediol, oleanolic acid, (R)-artabotriol, α-L-rhamnose, β-sitosterol and daucosterol (Takanori and Tomohiko, 2002; Yamamoto *et al.,* 2000; Zhang *et al.,* 2009).

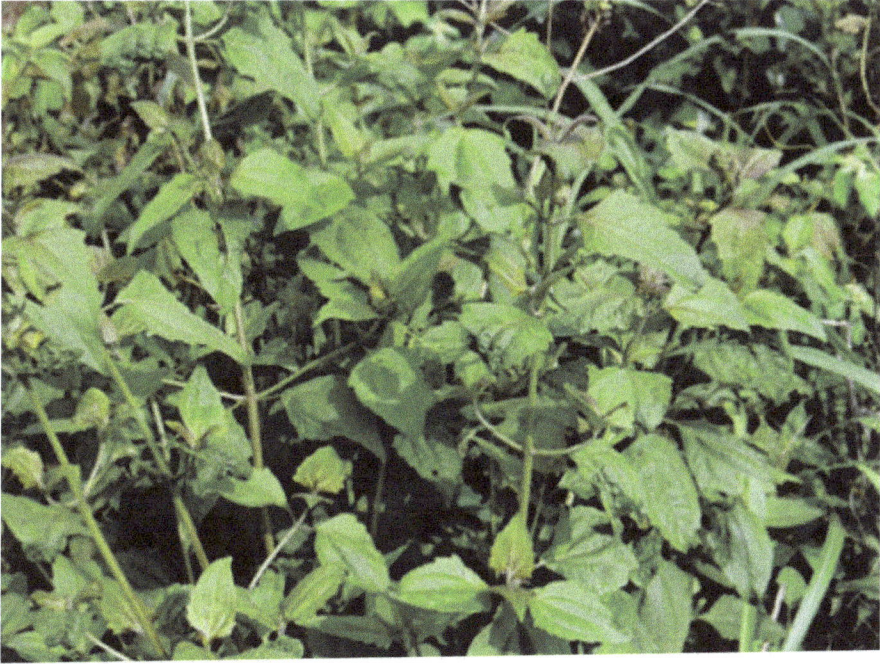

Family: Asteraceae

Botanical name: *Chromolaena odorata*

Common names: Siam weed

Local names: *Edo:* ebe-awolowo. *Igbo:* Igwulube. *Yoruba:* Ominira, Akintola

Parts used: leaves

Local uses: Leaf infusion is used to treat fever and diabetes. Prevents early miscarriage. Crushed fresh leaves and used to treat skin rashes. Leaves used as tonic and aids fertility. Siam weed extract accelerates hemostasis and wound healing (Akah,1990; Wongkrajang et al.,1990; Phan et al., 1998 and Phan, 2000).

Chemical constituents: Alkaloids, essential oil, Cardinol – pinene, limonene oxygenated sesqitespenoide flavonoids, oxalates, coumarin, saponin, tannins, vanillin

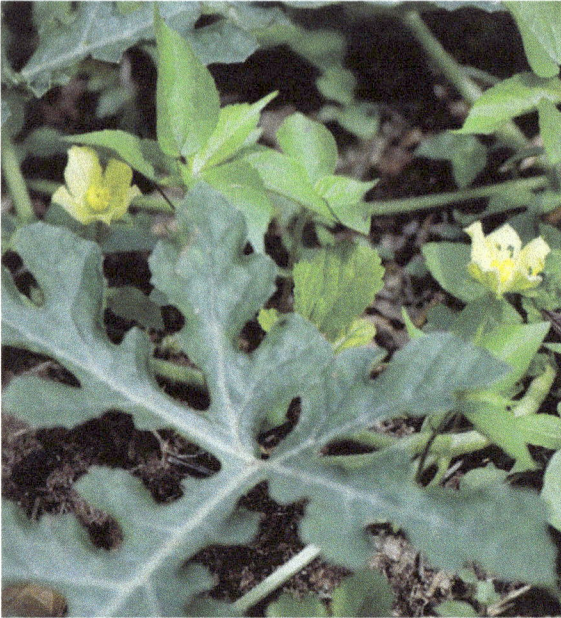

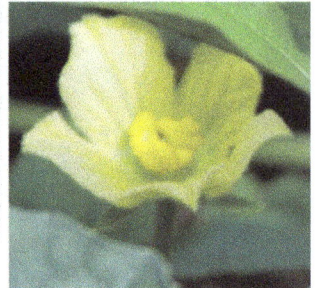

Family: Cucurbitaceae

Botanical name: Citrullus colocynthis

Common names: Wild gourd, melon

Local names: *Edo:* Ikpogi, Ogi. *Hausa:* Kwartowa. *Igbo:* Elili egusi, Ogili. *Yoruba;* Egusi baara

Parts used: Fruits, Leaf

Local uses: The fruit is eaten in large quantity as a remedy for urinary conditions. Seed shell powdered and mixed with palm oil is rubbed on skin to treat fungal infections. The melon shell is used to treat fungal infection on human skin. Topical *C. Colocynthis* also showed significant efficacy in treatment of patients with painful diabetic neuropathy; the application of a topical formulation of *C. colocynthis* fruit extract can decrease the pain and improve nerve function and quality of life in patients with painful diabetic neuropathy (Heydar, 2015). Colocynth has been widely used in folk medicine for centuries. Johann Weyer, in *De praestigiis daemonum* (1563), offers it as a cure for lycanthropy (Mora, 1991). Heydari, Mojtaba; Homayouni, Kaynoosh; Hashempur, Mohammad Hashem; Shams, Mesbah (2015).

Chemical Constituents: The oil content of the seeds is 17–19% (w/w), consisting of 67–73% linoleic acid, 10–16% oleic acid, 5–8% stearic acid, and 9–12% palmitic acid. The oil yield is about 400 l/hectare. In addition, the seeds contain a high amount of arginine, tryptophan, and the sulfurcontaining amino acids (Gurudeeban *et al.,* 2010 and Schafferman, 1998).

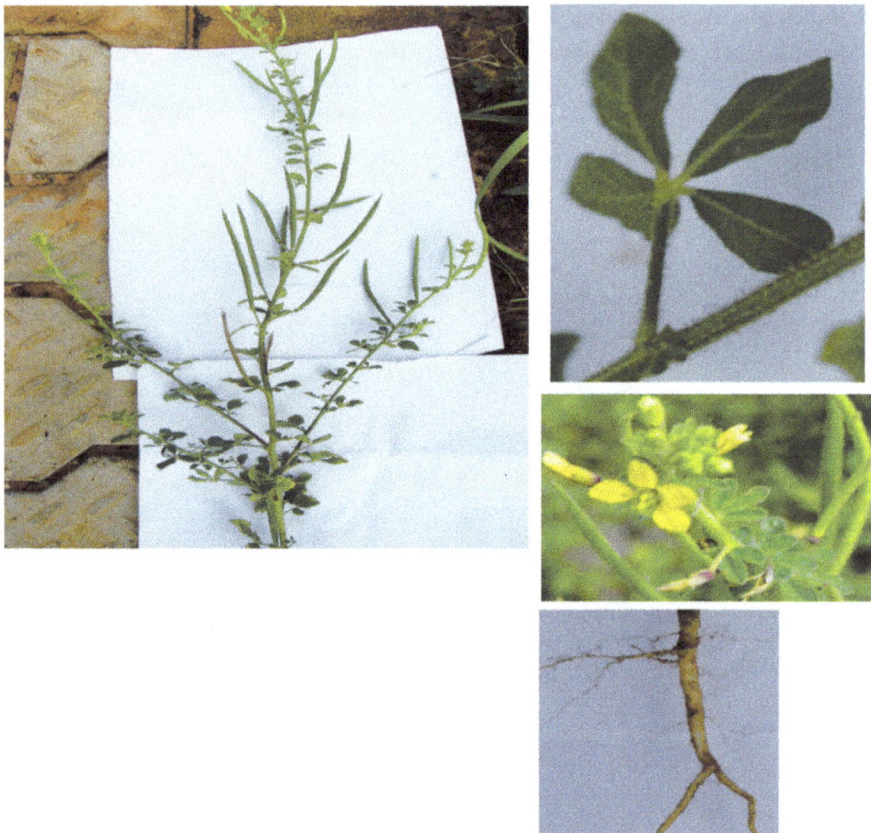

Family: Capparidaceae

Botanical name: *Cleome viscosa.*

Local uses: Anti-inflammatory and antipyretic (Tripti *et al.,* 2015 and Pari-maladevi *et al.,* 2003)

Chemical Constituents: Terpinoids, Coumarines, Flavonoids and Alkaloids (Jente, 1990 and Sharaf *et al.,* 1997).

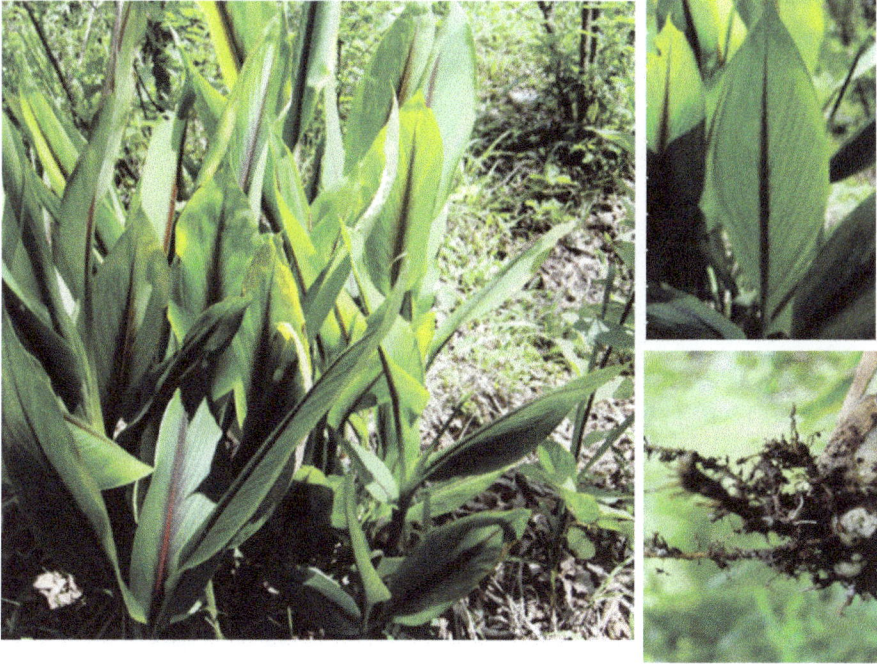

Botanical name: *Curcuma auriginosa*

Local uses: They are used to treat a range of conditions including colic, asthma and cough, obesity and rheumatism.

Chemical constituents: Sesquiterpenes, curcumenol, zedoarol, isocurcumenol, phytosterol mixtures containing stigmasterol and α-sitosterol (Saad, 2006).

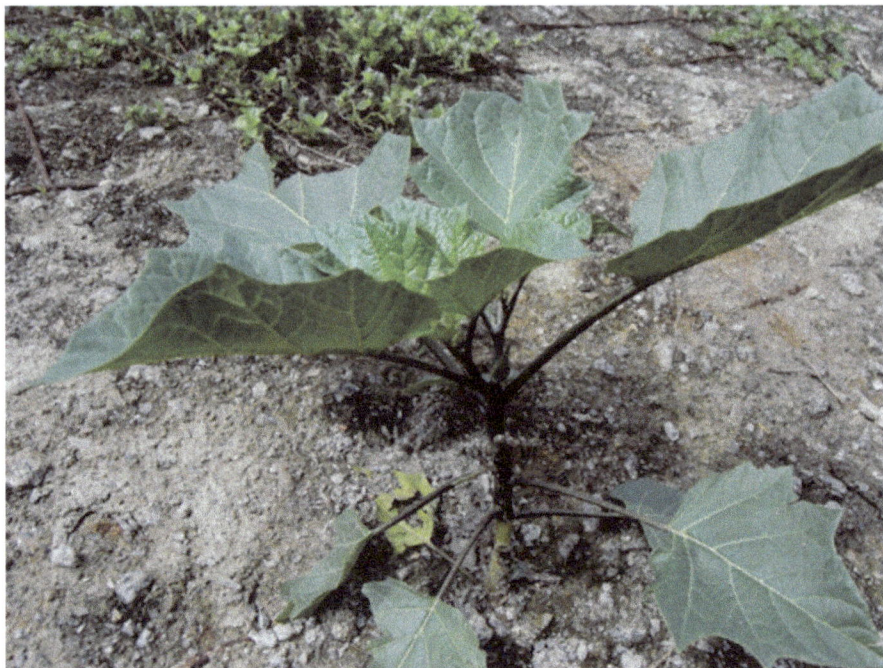

Botanical name: *Datura stramomium*

Local uses: The Zuni people once used datura as an analgesic to render patients unconscious while broken bones were set. The Chinese also used it as a form of anesthesia during surgery (Turner, 2009; Nellis and David, 1997).

Chemical constituents: All parts of Datura plants contain dangerous levels of the tropane alkaloids, atropine, hyoscyamine, and scopolamine, which are classified as deliriants, or anticholinergics. The risk of fatal overdose is high among uninformed users, and many hospitalizations occur amongst recreational users who ingest the plant for its psychoactive effects (Preissel and Hans-Georg, 2002).

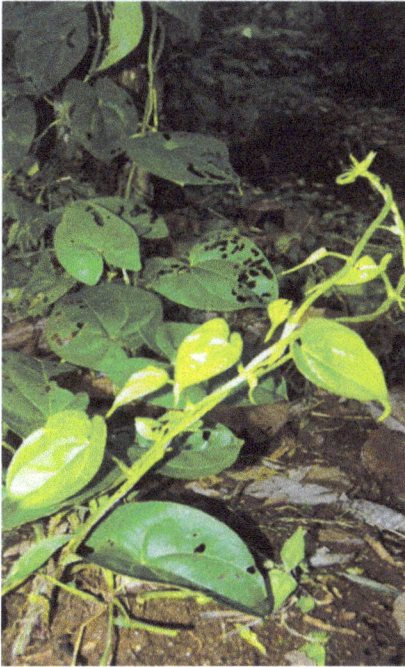

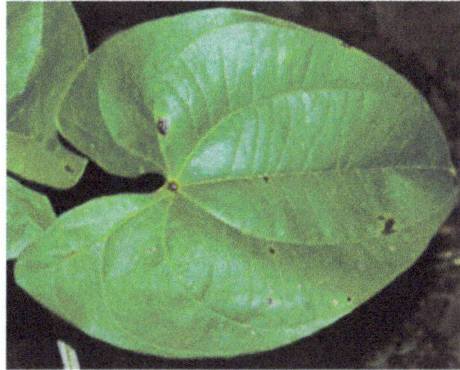

Family: Dioscoriaceae

Botanical name: *Dioscorea alata*

Common name: water yam or purple yam Local Names:

History: Dioscorea alata is native to Southeast Asia, as well as surrounding areas (Taiwan, Ryukyu Islands of Japan, Assam, lowland areas of Nepal, New Guinea, Christmas Island). It has moved from its native growth area and into the wild in many other places.

Local use: In folk medicine, *D. alata* has been used as a moderate laxative and vermifuge, and for fever, gonorrhea, leprosy, tumors, and inflamed hemorrhoids (Wanasundera and Ravindran, 1994).

Chemical constituents: The color of purple varieties is due to various anthocyanin pigments (Moriya, 2015).

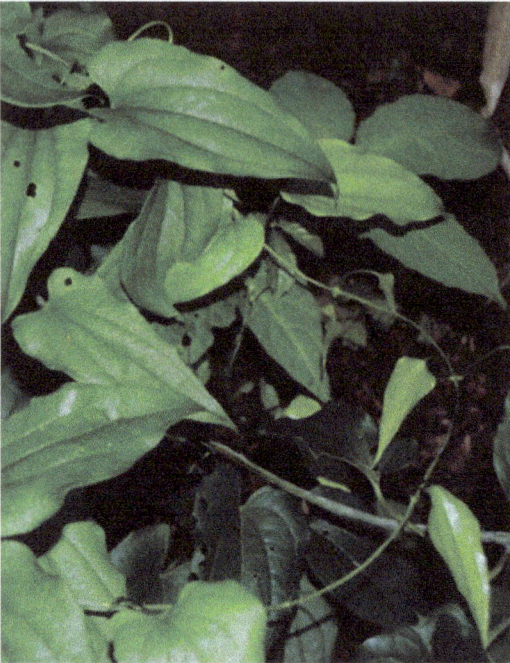

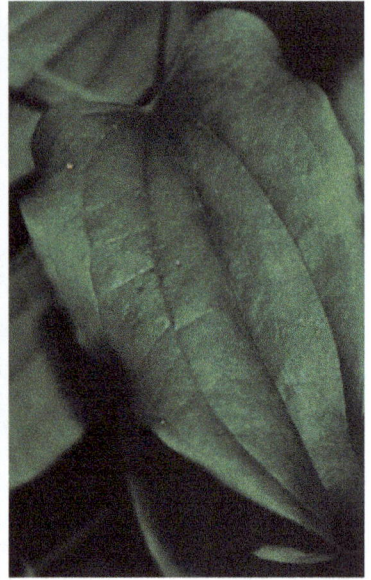

Family: *Dioscoriaceae*
Botanical name: Dioscorea cayenensis
Common name: Yellow yam

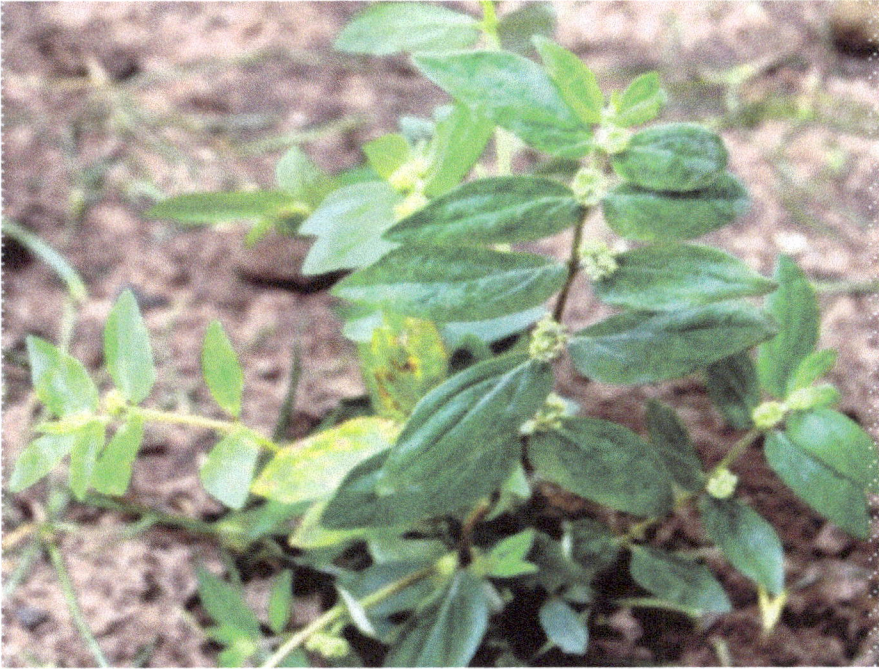

Family: Euphorbiaceae

Botanical name: *Euphorbia hirta*

Common names: Asthma plant, cat's hair, hairy spurge, Pills bearing spurge.

Parts used: Whole plant

Local uses: It is also used as a remedy for hay fever and catarrh. Leaves increase lactation in nursing mothers. The latex is used for conjunctivitis and ulcerated Cornea. E. hirta is used in the treatment of gastrointestinal disorders (diarrhoea, dysentery, intestinal parasitosis, etc.), bronchial and respiratory diseases (asthma, bronchitis, hay fever, etc.), and in conjunctivitis. Hypotensive and tonic properties are also reported in E. hirta. The aqueous extract exhibits anxiolytic, analgesic, antipyretic, and anti-inflammatory activities. The stem sap is used in the treatment of eyelid styes and a leaf poultice is used on swelling and boils (Galvez *et al.,* 1993).

Chemical constituents: shikmic acid, tinyatoxin, choline, camphol, and quercitol derivatives containing rhamnose and chtolphenolic acid (Sood, 2005).

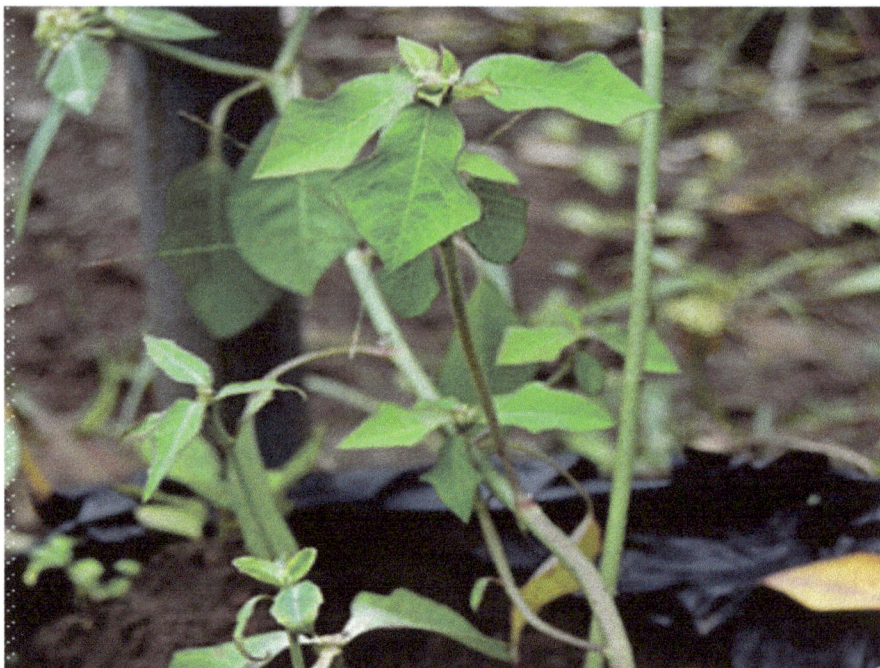

Family: Euphorbiaceae

Botanical name: *Euphorbia heterophylla*

Parts used: Whole plant

Local uses: Latex is used to treat insect bites. For the treatment of erysipelas cough, bronchial paroxysmal asthma, hay fever, catarrh. It is used as anti gonorrheal, for migraine and wartcures. A decoction or infusion of the stems and fresh or dried leaves is taken as a purgative and laxative to treat stomach-ache and constipation, and to expel intestinal worms

Chemical constituents: Flavonoid; kaempferol and quercetin (Singh and Kumar, 2013).

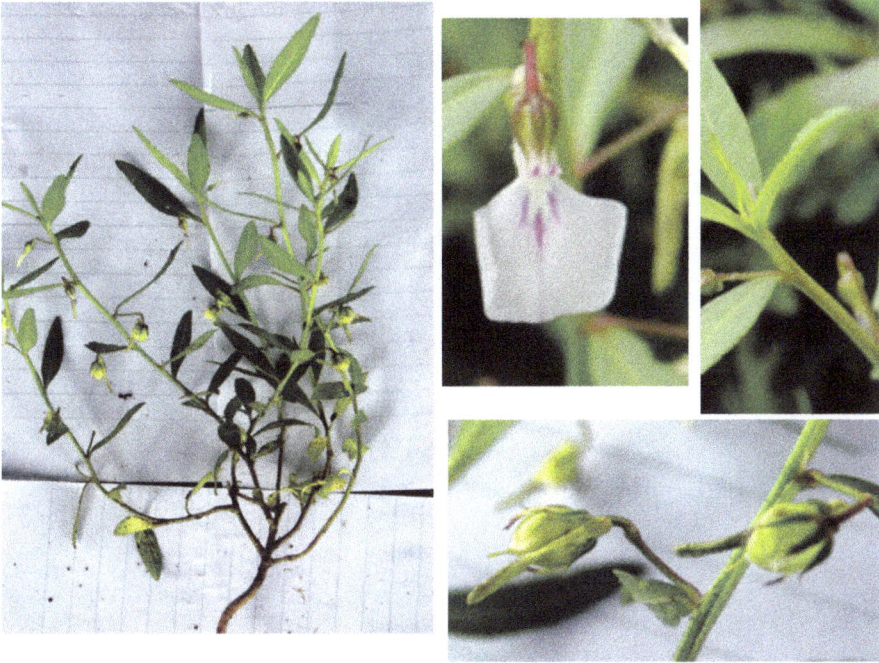

Family: *Violaceae*

Botanical name: *Hybanthus enneaspermus*

Common name: Humpback flower

History: This is a plant of coastal savannah, grassland, cultivated fields, barren lands and roadsides, and is often found growing on open grassland near the seashore. It is found widely in Africa and Madagascar, scattered in India, Sri Lanka, Indochina, south-east China, the Philippines, Borneo, East Java, New Guinea and the northern parts of Australia, and recently found in the Hengchun Peninsula of Taiwan

Local uses: In traditional medicines, the whole plant is considered to possess tonic, diuretic and demulcent properties. A decoction of the leaves and tender branches is used to sooth the skin, and these parts of the plant are also made into a cooling liniment for the head. Dried powderedleaves are used to treat asthma.

Chemical constituents: Alkaloids, terpenoids, saponins, flavonoids, Tannin, glycosides, phenols, steroids and reducing sugars.

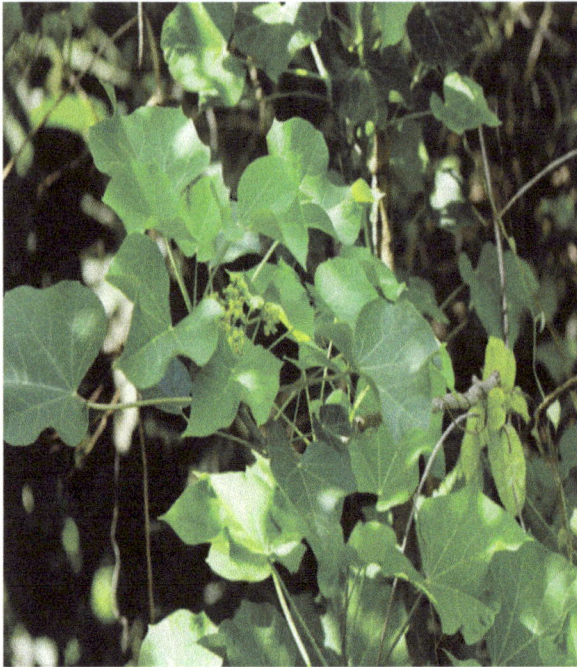

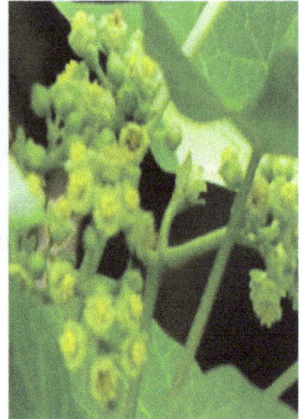

Family: Euphorbiaceae

Botanical name: *Jathropha curcas*

Common name: Barbados nut, physic nut

Local name: *Benin:* Oru-ebo-, ukpono. ***Igbo:*** Olulu-idu, Owulu-idu, Oluoyibo, Ochocho. ***Hausa:*** Dazugu, Biinida zugaga, Halallamai. ***Yoruba:*** Lapalapa, Botuje, Dodoromi, Lakose, Lobotuje, Olobutije, seluju, Serise

Local Uses: Abortifacient, antibacterial and analgesic.

Chemical Constituents: *J. curcas* also contains compounds such as trypsin inhibitors, phytate, saponins and a type of lectin (Makkar *et al.*, 2008 and Martínez-Herrera *et al.*, 2012).

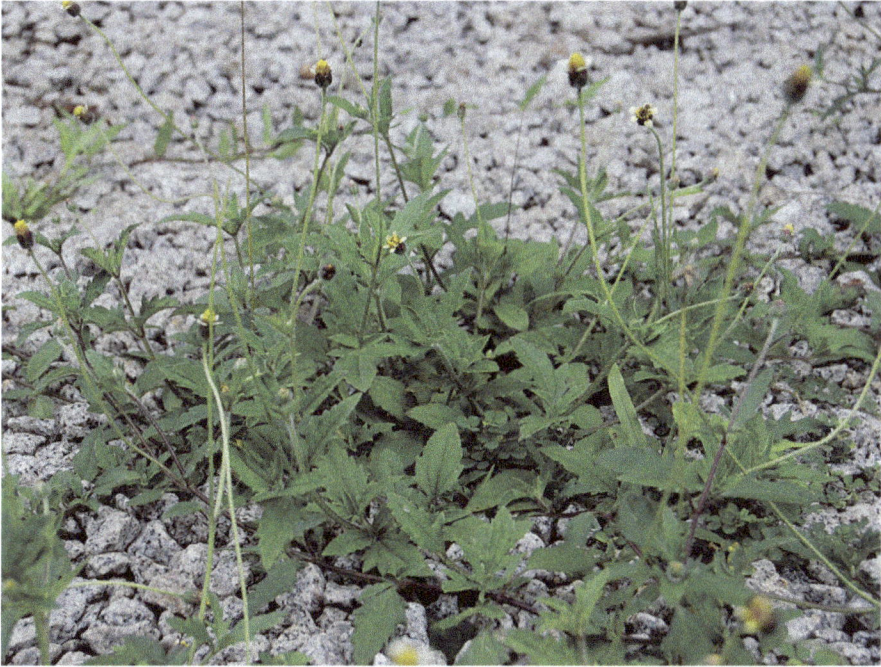

Family: Asteraceae

Botanical name: *Tridax procumbens*

Common name: Coatbuttons or tridax daisy

History: It is native to the tropical Americas, but it has been introduced to tropical, subtropical, and mild temperate regions worldwide.

References

Aboushoer, M.I., Fathy, H.M., Abdel-Kader, M.S., Goetz, G., Omar, A.A.(2010) Terpenes and flavonoids from an Egyptian collection of Cleome droserifolia. Advances in Applied Science Research, 2 (3): 219-226

Akah P. A. (1990). Mechanism of hemostatic activity of Eupatorium odoratum. International Journal of Crude Drug Research,28 (4):253–256.

Amabye TG (2015). Evaluation of Physiochemical, Phytochemical, Antioxidant and Antimicrobial Screening Parameters of Amaranthus spinosus Leaves. Nat Prod Chem Res, 4:199.

BMC Complementary and Alternative Medicine Volume 7 http://www biomedcentral.com.

Bown. D. (1995). Encyclopaedia of Herbs and their Uses. Publication. Dorling Kindersley, London.

Burkil. H. M. (1985-2004). The Useful Plants of West Tropical Africa. Royal Botanic Gardens Publisher Kew.

Burkill, H.M., 1995. The useful plants of West Tropical Africa. 2nd Edition. Volume 3, Families J–L. Royal Botanic Gardens, Kew, Richmond, United Kingdom. 857 pp.

Chopra, B (1933). Further notes on Crustaceae Decapoda in the Indian Museum. V, On Eutrichocheles Modestus (Herbst): Family Axiidae. R

Chopra, R. N., Nayar. S. L. and Chopra. I. C. (1986). Glossary of Indian Medicinal Plants (Including the Supplement). Council of Scientific and Industrial Research, New Delhi. Cleome viscosa., Phytochemistry29, 2: 666-667

Duke, J.A. (1985). CRC Handbook of Medicinal Herbs. 677 pp. Boca Raton, Florida: CRC Press.

Duke, J. A. and Ayensu. E. S. (1985). Medicinal Plants of China Reference Publications, Inc. ISBN 0-917256-20-4

Emmanuel, E. E., Imo, E. J. and Paul, S.T (2015). Phytochemical Composition, Antimicrobial and Antioxidant Activities of Leaves and Tubers of Three Caladium Species. International Journal of Medicinal Plants and Natural Products, 1(2): 24-30.

Galvez, J., Zarzuelo A, Crespo ME, Lorente MD, Ocete MA, Jimenez J. (1993). Antidiarrhoeal activity of Euphorbia hirta extract and isolation of an active flavanoid constituent. Planta Med., 59:333– 36.

Grenand, P., Moretti, C. and H. Jacquemin. 1987. Pharmacopées Tradition-nelles en Guyane: Créoles, Palikur, Wayapi. 569 pp. Paris: Editions de l'ORSTOM

Grindlay, D., Reynolds, T. (1986). The aloe vera phenomenon: a review of the properties and modern uses of the leaf parenchyma gel. J. Ethnopharmacol, 16(2-3):117-151.

Gurudeeban, S.; Satyavani K.; Ramanathan T. (2010). "Bitter Apple (Citrullus colocynthis): An Overview of Chemical Composition and Biomedical Potentials". Asian Journal of Plant Sciences. 9 (7): 394–401.

Hamid, A. A., Aiyelaagbe O. O., Ahmed R. N., Usman L. A. and Adebayo S. A. (2001). Preliminary Phytochemistry, Antibacterial and Anti-fungal Properties of extracts of Asystasia gangetica Linn T. Andersongrown in Nigeria

Heckel, E. 1897. Les Plantes Médicinales et Toxiques de la Guya Heide, L. (2006). Artemisinin in traditional tea preparations of Artemisia annua. Trans R Soc Trop Med Hyg;100(8):802. 16701762

Hemen, D. and Lalita L. (2012). A review of anthraquinones isolated from Cassia species and their applications. Indian Journal of Natural Products and Resources, 3 (3): 291-319.

Henry, R (1979). An updated review of aloe vera. Cosmetics and Toiletries P:94: 42.

Hsu, E. (2006). The history of qing hao in the Chinese materia medica. Trans R Soc Trop Med Hyg; 100(6):505-508. 16566952

Igboh, M. Ngozi, Ikewuchi C. Jude and C. Catherine, 2009. Chemical Profile of Chromolaena odorata L. (King and Robinson) Leaves. Pakistan Journal of Nutrition, 8: 521-524.

Jaccoud, R.J.S. 1961. Contribuição para o estudo formacognóstico do Ageratum conyzoides L. Rev. Bras. Farm. 42(11/12):177–97.

Jente, R., Jakupovic J. Olatunji G.A. (1990), A cembranoid diterpene from K. Bairwa, A. Srivastava, and S. M. Jachak, (2014). Quantitative analysis of Boeravinones in the roots of Boerhaavia diffusa by UPLC/ PDA, Phytochemical Analysis.

Kissmann, G. and D. Groth. (1993). Plantas infestantes e nocivas. Basf Brasileira, São Paulo.

Klayman DL (1985). Quinghasosu (artemisinin), an antimalarial drug from China. Science, 228: 1049-1055.

Kokwaro, JO (1976). Medicinal plants of East Africa, General Printers Ltd, Kenya, Pp. 12.

Lans CA (2006). "Ethnomedicines used in Trinidad and Tobago for urinary problems and diabetes mellitus". J Ethnobiol Ethnomed. 2: 45. PMC 1624823. PMID 17040567. doi:10.1186/1746-4269-2-45

Leung AY, Foster S (1980.). Encyclopedia of Common Natural Ingredients Used in Food, Drugs, and Cosmetics. New York, NY: J Wiley and Sons

Li, Y. and Wu, Y. L. (1998) How Chinese scientists discovered qinghaosu (artemisinin) and developed its derivatives? What are the future perspectives? Med Trop (Mars), 58(3 Suppl):9-12. 10212890

Liu H, Chou GX, Guo YL, Ji LL, Wang JM, et al. (2010). Norclerodane diterpenoids from rhizomes of Dioscorea bulbifera Phytochemistry 71: 1174-1180.

Liu H, Chou GX, Wu T, Guo YL, Wang SC, et al. (2009) Steroidal sapogenins and glycosides from the rhizomes of Dioscorea bulbifera. J Nat Prod 72: 1964-1968.

Lommen, W. J., Schenk, E., Bouwmeester, H. J., and Verstappen, F.W. (2006). Trichome dynamics and artemisinin accumulation during development and senescence of Artemisia annua leaves. Planta Med, 72(4):336-345. 16557475

Makkar, H.P.S., Francis, G., Becker, K. 2008. Protein concentrate from Jatropha curcas screw-pressed seed cake and toxic and antinutritional factors in protein concentrate. Journal of Science of Food and Agriculture 88: 1542-1548.

Martínez-Herrera, J., Jiménez-Martínez, C., Martínez Ayala, A., Garduño-Siciliano, L., Mora-Escobedo, R., Dávila-Ortiz, G., Chamorro-Cevallos, G., Makkar, H.P.S., Francis, G., Becker, K. 2012. Evaluation of the nutritional quality of non-toxic kernel flour from Jatropha curcas L. in rats. Journal of Food Quality 35:152-158.

May, A.F. 1982. Surinaams Kruidenboek (Sranan Oso Dresi). 80 pp.

Paramaribo, Surinam: Vaco; and Zutphen, The Netherlands: De Walburg Pers

Ming, L.C. (1999). Ageratum conyzoides: A tropical source of medicinal and agricultural products. In Janick, J. Perspectives on new crops and new uses. Alexandria VA: ASHS Press. pp. 469–473.

Mora, George; Kohl, Benjamin G.; Midelfort, Erik; Bacon, Helen, eds. (1991). Witches, devils, and doctors in the Renaissance: Johann Weyer, De praestigiis daemonum. Translated by John Shea Binghamton: Medieval and Renaissance Texts and Studies. p. 343

Moriya C, Hosoya T, Agawa S, Sugiyama Y, Kozone I, Shin-Ya K (2015). New acylated anthocyanins from purple yam and their antioxidant activity. Biosci Biotechnol Biochem. 79 (9): 1484–92

Nellis, D. W. (1997). Poisonous Plants and Animals of Florida and the Caribbean Pineapple Press. p. 238. ISBN 978-1-56164-111-6. Nelson, K. M. Dahlin, J. L., Bisson, J. (2017). The Essential Medicinal Chemistry of Curcumin: Miniperspectiv. Journal of Medicinal Chemistry.60 (5): 1620–1637

Odeja, O., Ogwuche, C. E., Elemike, E. E. (2017). Clin. Phytosci. 2: 12. https://doi.org/10.1186/s40816-016-0027-2

OKO, O. O. K. and Agiang, E. A. (2001). Phytochemical activities of Aspilia africana leaf using different extractants. Indian Journal of Animal Sciences 81 (8): 814–818.

Oluyemi, K. A., Okwuonu, U.C., Baxter, D. G. & Oyesola Tolulope, O., (2007). Toxic Effects of Methanolic Extract of Aspilia africana Leaf on the Estrous Cycle and Uterine Tissues of Wistar Rats" Int. J. Morphol., 25(3):609-614.

Oyetayo V.O. (2007). Comparative Studies of the Phytochemical and Antimicrobial Properties of the Leaf, Stem and Tuber of Anchomanes difformis. Journal of Pharmacology and Toxicology, 2: 407-410. Goode, P. M. (1989). FAO Food and nutrition paper 42(1), Edible plants of Uganda: the value of wild and cultivated plants as food.

Parimaladevi, B., Boominathan, R. and Mandal, S.C. (2003) Evaluation of antipyretic potential of Cleome viscosa Linn. (Capparidaceae) extract in rats. Journal of Phan T. T., Allen J., Hughes M. A., Cherry G. and Wojnarowska F. (2000). Upregulation of adhesion complex proteins and fibronectin by human keratinocytes treated with an aqueous extract from the leaves of Chromolaena odorata (Eupolin)," European Journal of Dermatology, vol. 10, no. 7, pp. 522–527,

Phan T. T., Hughes M. A., and Cherry G. W. (1998). Enhanced proliferation of fibroblasts and endothelial cells treated with an extract of the leaves of Chromolaena odorata (Eupolin), an herbal remedy for treating wounds," Plastic and Reconstructive Surgery, vol. 101, no. 3, pp. 756–765.

Phan, V. T. (2002). [Artemisinine and artesunate in the treatment of malaria in Vietnam (1984-1999)]. Bull Soc Pathol Exot 95(2):86-88. 12145966

Preissel, Ulrike & Hans-Georg Preissel (2002). Brugmansia and Datura: Angel's Trumpets and Thorn Apples. Firefly Books. pp. 124–125.

R. Govindarajan, M. Vijayakumar, and P. Pushpangadan (2005). Antioxidant approach to disease management and the role of 'Rasayana' herbs of Ayurveda, Journal of Ethnopharmacology, vol. 99, no. 2, pp. 165–178, Rivera-Pastrana DM, Yahia EM, González-Aguilar GA (2010). Phenolic and carotenoid profiles of papaya fruit (Carica papaya L.) and their contents under low temperature storage. J Sci Food Agric. 90 (14): 2358–65.

Rossetto MR, Oliveira do Nascimento JR, Purgatto E, Fabi JP, Lajolo FM, Cordenunsi BR (2008). Benzylglucosinolate, enzylisothiocyanate, and myrosinase activity in papaya fruit during development and ripening. J Agric Food Chem., 56 (20): 9592–9.

Saad M. S. (2006) Phytochemical Constituents and Biological Activity of Curcuma Aeruginosa Roxb., C. Ochrorhiza Val. and Andrographis Asculata Nees. Masters thesis, Universiti Putra Malaysia.

Schafferman, D.; Beharav A.; Shabelsky E.; Yaniv Z (1998). Evaluation of Citrullus colocynthis, a desert plant native in Israel, as a potential source of edible oil. Journal of Arid Environments. 40 (4): 431–43

Schmelzer, G.H. & Gurib-Fakim, A. (2008). Plant Resources of Tropical Africa 11(1). Medicinal plants 1. PROTA Foundation, Wageningen, Netherlands / Backhuys Publishers, Leiden, Netherlands / CTA, Wageningen, Netherlands. 791 pp.

Seigler DS, Pauli GF, Nahrstedt A, Leen R (2002). Cyanogenic allosides and glucosides from Passiflora edulis and Carica papaya. Phytochemistry, 60 (8): 873–82.

Sharaf M., El-Ansari M.A., Saleh N.A.M .(1997) Flavonoids of four Cleomeand three Capparis species. Biochemical Systematics and Ecology. 25,(2): 161–166.

Simon KV, Charles DJ, Wood KV, Heinstein P (1990). Germplasm variation in artemisinin content of Artemisia annua L. using an alternative from crude plant extract. J. Nat. Prod., 3: 157-160 Singh G, Kumar P. (2013). Phytochemical study and screening for antimicrobial activity of flavonoids of Euphorbia hirta .Int J Appl Basic Med Res. 2013 Jul;3(2):111-6.

Sood SK, Bhardwaj R, Lakhanpal TN (2005). India: Scientific Publishers. Ethnic Indian Plants in cure of diabetes.

Supratman U; Fujita T; Akiyama K; et al. (2001). "Anti-tumor promoting activity of bufadienolides from Kalanchoe pinnata and K. daigremontiana x tubiflora" (PDF). Biosci. Biotechnol. Biochem. 65 (4): 947–9. PMID 11388478. doi:10.1271/ bbb.65.947.

Supratman U; Fujita T; Akiyama K; Hayashi H (2000). "New insecticidal bufadienolide, bryophyllin C, from Kalanchoe pinnata" (PDF). Biosci. Biotechnol. Biochem. 64 (6): 1310–2

Takanori Sugimoto, Tomohiko Fujii et al. (2002). Syntheses of novel photoaffinity probes for bioorganic studies on nyctinasty of leguminous plants. Tetrahedron Letters, 43 (37):6529-6532

Tanaka, Yoshitaka; Van Ke, Nguyen (2007). Edible Wild Plants of Vietnam: The Bountiful Garden. Thailand: Orchid Press. p. 22

Tang Z, Zhou Y, Zeng Y, Zang S, He P, et al. (2006) Capillary electrophoresis of the active ingredients of Dioscorea bulbifera L. and its medicinal preparations. Chromatographia 63: 617-62

Teponno RB, Tapondjou AL, Gatsing D, Djoukeng JD, Abou-Mansour Et al. (2006) Bafoudiosbulbins A, and B, two anti-salmonellal clerodane diterpenoids from Dioscorea bulbifera L. var sativa. Phytochemistry 67: 1957-1963.

Titanji, V.P.; Zofou, D.; Ngemenya, M.N. (2008). The Antimalarial Potential of Medicinal Plants Used for the Treatment of Malaria in Cameroonian Folk Medicine.African Journal of Traditional, Complementary and Alternative Medicines. 5 (3): 302–321.

Tripti J., Neeraj K. and Preeti K., (2015) A Review on Cleome viscosa: Anendogenous Herb of Uttarakhand. Inter. J. Pharma Res.& Rev; 4(7):25-31.

Turner, Matt W. (2009). Remarkable Plants of Texas: Uncommon Accounts of Our Common Natives. University of Texas Press. p. 209. ISBN 978-0-292-71851-7.

Wanasundera JP, Ravindran G (1994). Nutritional assessment of yam (Dioscorea alata) tubers. Plant Foods Hum Nutr. 46 (1): 33–9.

Williams C (2013). Medicinal plants in Australia volume 4: an antipodean apothecary, Rosenberg Publishing Science 552: 437- 44.

Wongkrajang Y., Muagklum S., Peungvicha P., Jaiarj P., and Opartkiattikul N., (1990). Eupatorium odoratum linn: an enhancer of hemostasis," Mahidol University Journal of Pharmaceutical Sciences, vol. 17, pp. 9–13, www.arcjournals.org

Yamamoto M, Shimura S, Itoh Y et al. (200). Anti-obesity effects of lipase inhibitor CT-II, an extract from edible herbs, Nomame Herba, on rats fed a high-fat diet. International Journal of Obesity, 24 (6):758-764

Zhang, W., Zhang J., and Li, R. (2009). Inhibitory Effect of Ethanol Extract of Cassia mimosoides Linn. on Dimethylnitrosamine- induced Hepatic Fibrosis in Rats. Traditional Chinese Drug Research & Clinical Pharmacology

Chapter 6

Grasses

Grasses are mostly herbaceous monocotyledon plants (aside *Bambusa spp.*) with jointed stems and sheathed leaves. They are usually upright, cylindrical, with alternating leaves. They have roots which in some cases are modified into rhizomes or stolons. Their inflorescence is differentiated into the panicle, spike, and raceme.

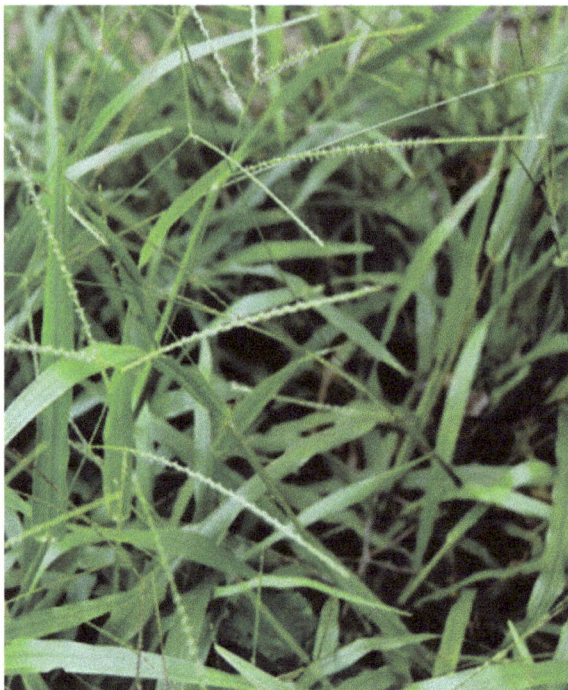

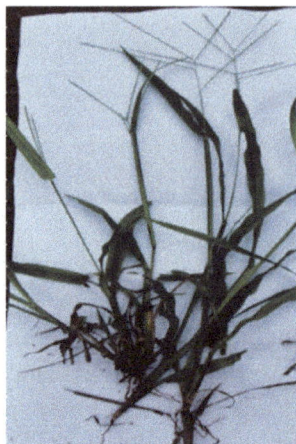

Family: Poaceae

Botanical name: *Axonopus compressus*

Common name: Broadleaf carpet grass, lawn grass

Local name: *Yoruba:* Idi

History: Blanket grass (*Axonopus compressus*) is a robust creeping perennial grass that forms dense mats. Foliage generally reaches up to 15 cm high and flowering culms up to 30-45 cm high. It is shallow-rooted, shortly rhizomatous with slender elongate and branched stolons that root at the nodes. Leaf blades are shiny, flat, folded, lanceolate, 4-15 cm long and 2.5-15 mm broad. Flowering culms are erect and laterally compressed. They bear racemose panicles. There are generally 2-3 racemes, although up to 5 is possible. The 2 upper racemes are paired and borne on a slender peduncle; they are generally one-sided. The secondary racemes usually remain hidden in the sheath.

Local uses: Blanket grass isused as green forage by traditional rabbit raisers in Central Java during both wet and the dry season (Prawirodigdo, 1985).

Chemical constituents: Crude protein is generally low. A high content of non-structural carbohydrates has also been reported, which may explain the high in vitro digestibility observed in some cases (Samarakoon *et al.,* 1990).

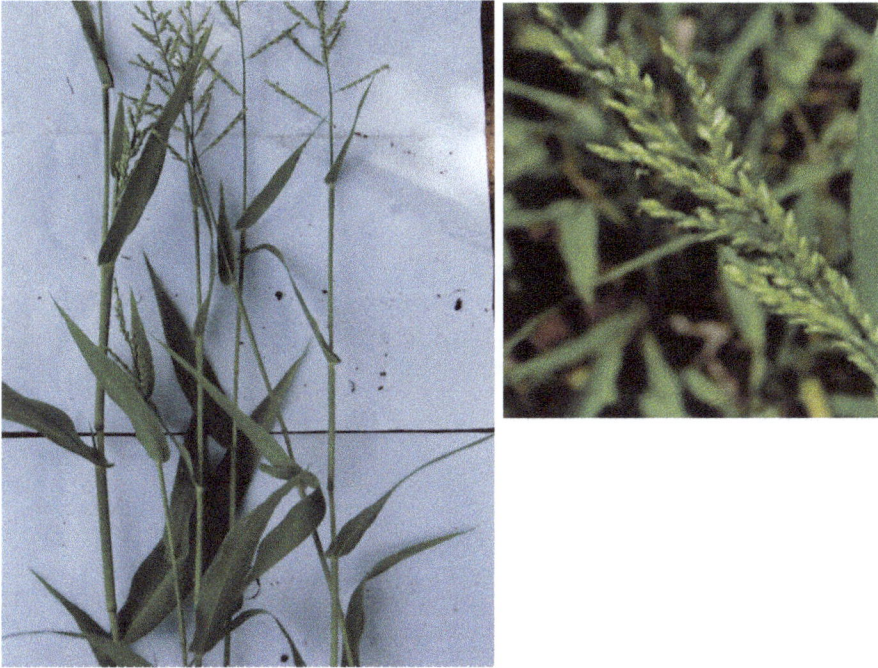

Family: Poaceae

Botanical name: *Brachiaria nigropedata*

History: *Brachiaria nigropedata* is a perennial grass belonging to the grass family (Poaceae). It is native to Southern Africa the tropical regions of South Africa and East Africa. Brachiaria nigropedata is used as fodder grass in Namibia (Rothauge, 2014).

Local uses: Ashes from the whole plant are used as a treatment against snake bite, Brachiaria, Urochloa (Gramineae-Paniceae) in Malesia. (Veld-kamp, 1996). The rhizomes are diuretic. A paste made from the rhizome is used in the treatment of kidney problems.

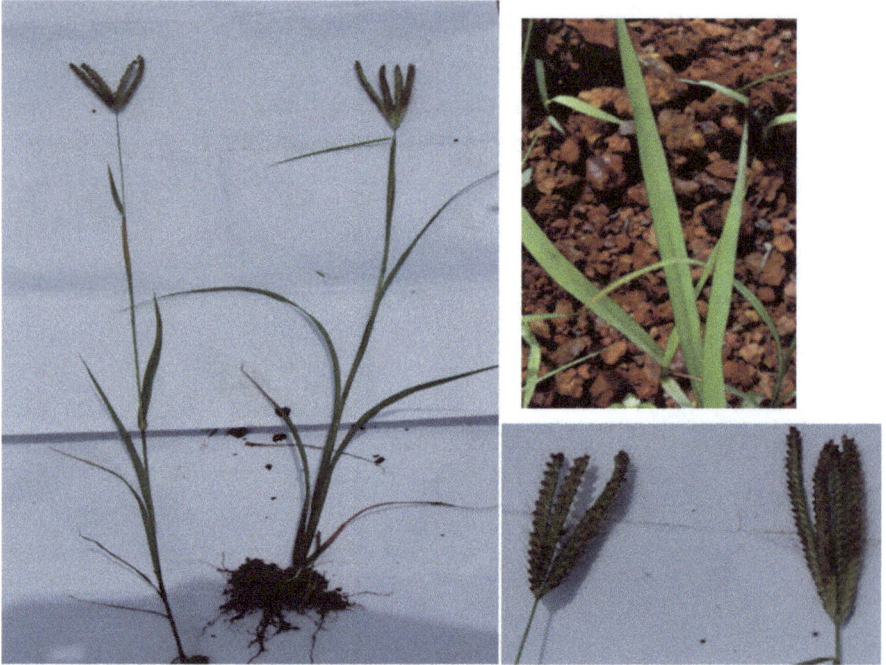

Family: Poaceae

Botanical name: *Chloris pilosa*

Common name: Windmill grass or finger grass.

Local name: *Yoruba:* Eéran

History: Chloris is a widespread genus of plants in the grass family, know generally as windmill grass or finger grass. The genus is found worldwide, but especially in the tropical and subtropical regions, and more often in the Southern Hemisphere. The species are variable in morphology, but in general the plants are less than half a meter in height. They bear inflorescences shaped like umbels, with several plumes lined with rows of spikelets.

Chemical constituents: Aqueous extract of leaves yielded phytosterols, flavonoids, tannins, phenols, carbohydrates, proteins and amino acids.

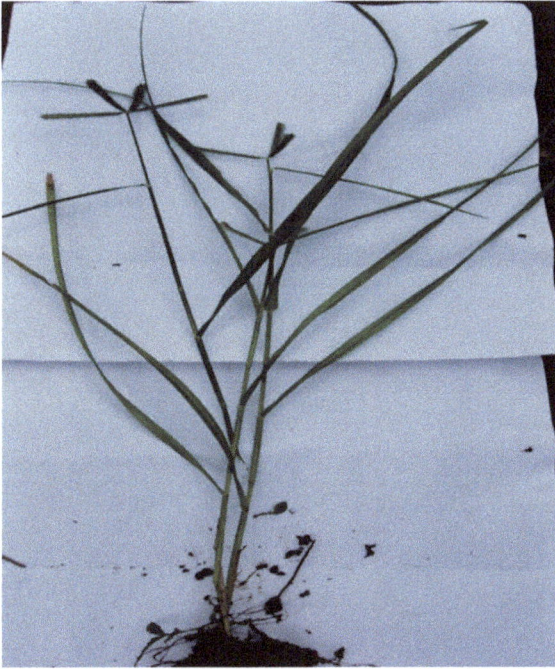

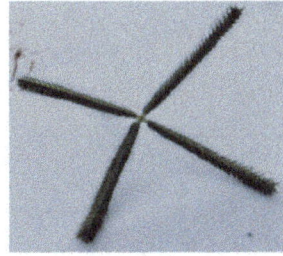

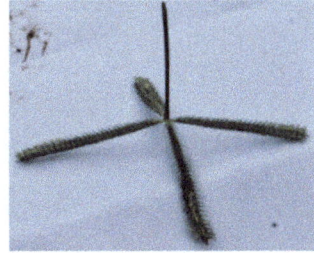

Family: Poaceae

Botanical name: *Dactyloctenium aegyptium*

Common name: Crowfoot grass, Indian wheat

Local name: *Hausa:* Kutukku

History: Coast button grass is a glaucous annual with culms up to 70cm high, not stoloniferous, but often rooting from the lower nodes. The plant can form a mat with short underground stems. The seed is sometimes harvested from the wild for food, but generally only in times of scarcity. The plant also has local medicinal uses Ruffo, Birnie, & Tengnas, (2002).

Local uses: The whole plant is used in a decoction to remedy lumbago. An infusion of the leaves, mixed with the seeds of *Cajanus cajan*, is used to accelerate childbirth. A decoction of the leaves, combined with *Scoparia dulcis*, is used as a remedy for dysentery. DeFilipps, Maina, & Crepin, J. 1984).

Chemical constituents: The plant is rich in cyanogenetic glucosides at certain stages of growth times.

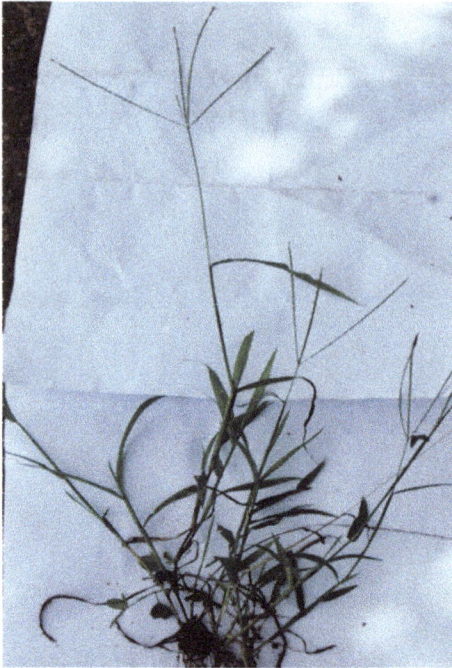

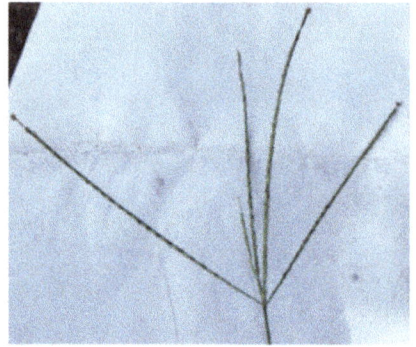

Family: Poaceae

Botanical name: *Digitaria spp*

History: Digitaria is an annual growing to 0.5 m (1ft 8in) at a fast rate.

It is hardy to zone (UK) 7. It is in flower from August to September. The flowers are hermaphrodite (have both male and female organs) and are pollinated by Wind. Suitable for: light (sandy) and medium (loamy) soils. Suitable pH: acid, neutral and basic (alkaline) soils. It cannot grow in the shade. It prefers moist soil.

Local uses: A decoction of the plant is used in the treatment of gonorrhoea. A folk remedy for cataracts and debility, it is also said to be emetic. Duke.J. A. and Ayensu. E. S. Medicinal Plants of China Reference Publications, Inc. ISBN 0-917256-20-4 (1985-00-00).

Chemical constituents: Crabgrass harvest may potentially yield more than 15% crude protein and 60% total digestible nutrients (TDN). Studies on chemical composition have yielded (%DM) crude protein 12.0-19.2%, total condensed tannin 0.12-0.20%, soluble sugar 5.7-6.3%, NDF 44.2-52.3%, OMD 71.2-76.4%.. Study on digestibility (IVDMD) and metabolizing energy (ME) study yielded 59.3% and 7.99% at early bloom, respectively, and 42.6% and 5.52% at maturity, respectively (Orskov, E.R. 1982 Protein Nutrition in Ruminants. Academic Press, London).

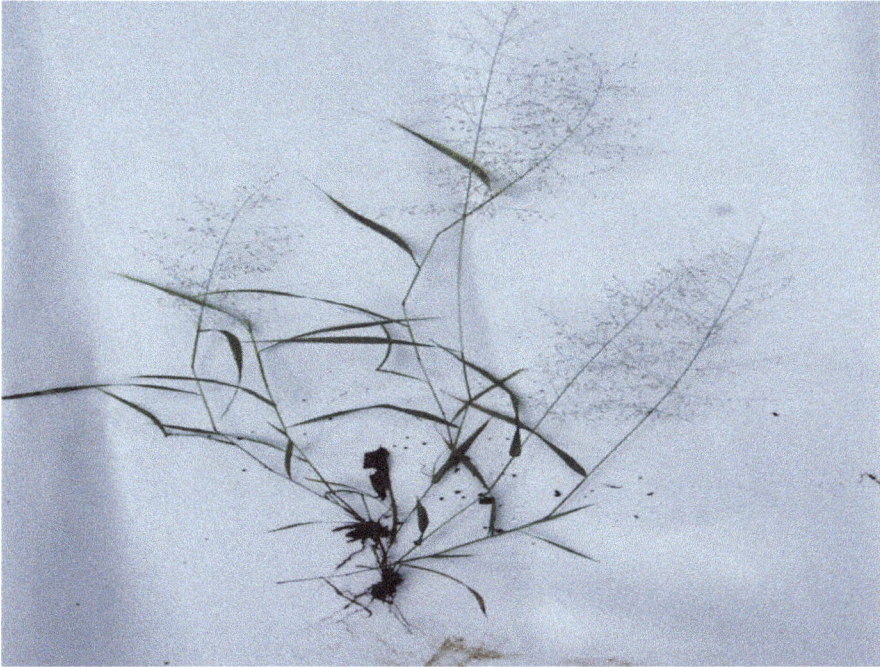

Family: Poaceae

Botanical name: *Eragrostis tenella*

Common name: Love grass

History: *Eragrostis tenella* is a small densely tufted annual grass, with variable size, usually not much more than 50cm high. Clums glabrous, spindly, the nodes at the base, may be ramified or not. Leaves up to 10cm long. Inflorescence usually with many slender spreading branches. (Galinato, Moody, Piggin, 1999).

Local uses: Seed Sometimes eaten as a cereal, it is said to be nutritious. The seed is small and fiddly to utilize—it is most commonly seen as a famine food, used when nothing better is available. The Useful Plants of West Tropical Africa. Burkil. H. M.(1985 – 2004)

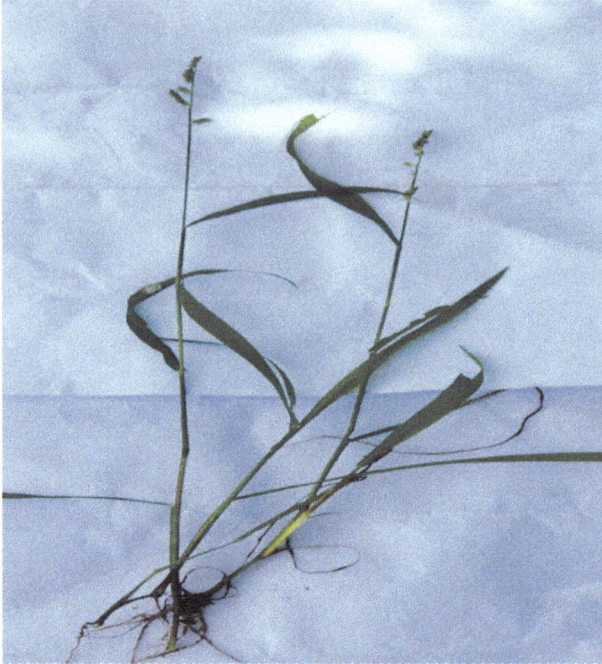

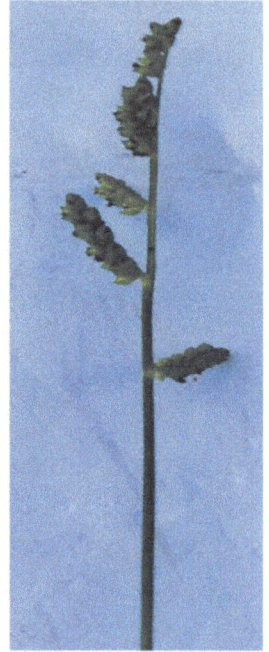

Family: Poaceae

Botanical name: *Echonochloa spp*

History: Barnyard millet is an annual plant that can succeed in a wide range of environments from the temperate zone to the tropics. It can be found at elevations up to 2,500 metres. It grows best in areas where annual daytime temperatures are within the range 17-30°c but can tolerate 2-40°c It prefers a mean annual rainfall in the range 700-1,100mm, but tolerates 310-2,500mm. An easily grown plant, it is adapted to nearly all types of wet places, and is often a common weed in paddy fields, roadsides, cultivated areas, and fallow fields.

Local uses: Reported to be preventative and tonic, barnyard grass is a folk remedy for treating carbuncles, haemorrhages, sores, spleen trouble, cancer and wounds. Handbook of Energy Crops Duke. J.(1983).

Chemical Constituents: Nitrate. Duke. J.(1983).

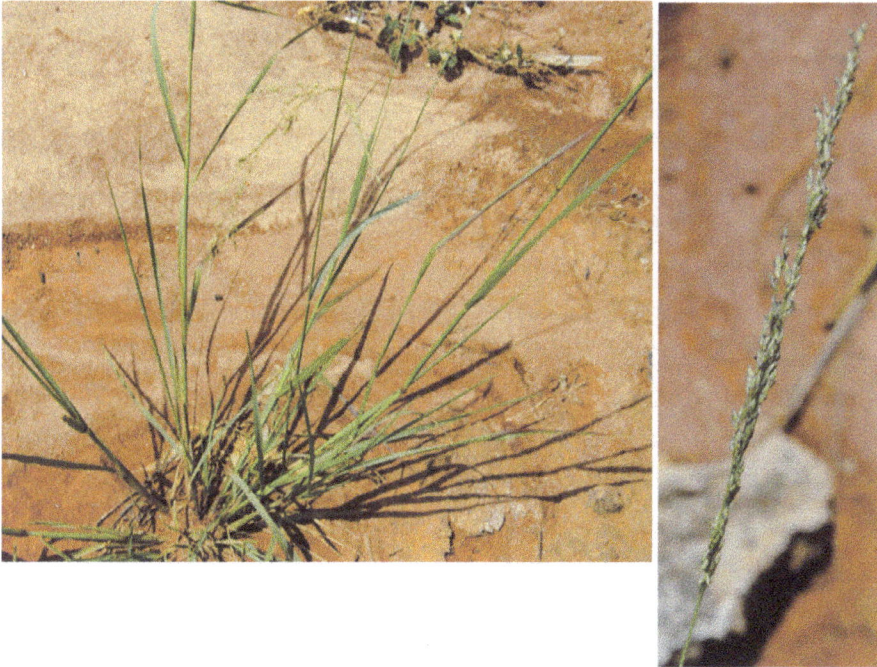

Family: Poaceae

Botanical name: *Eragrostis tremula*

History: Eragrostis tremula is a loosely clump-forming, annual to perennial grass with erect, usually unbranched culms up to 100cm tall. These culms have attractive trembling panicles. The plant is harvested from the wild for local use as a food and source of material. The Useful Plants of West Tropical Africa. Burkil. H. M. (1985 – 2004).

Local uses: The culms, bundled together, are used as hand-brooms for idoor use. The culms may also be used for thatching, and are woven together to make mats and cordage.

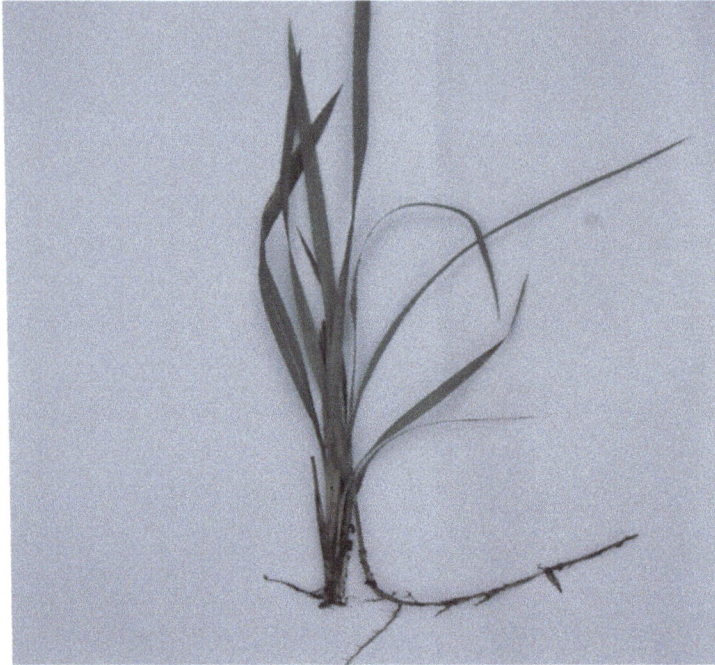

Family: Poaceae

Botanical name: *Imperata cylindrical*

Common name: Spear grass, Blady grass, Congo grass

Local name: *Igbo:* Atta. *Yoruba:* Ekan

History: Cogon grass is a perennial grass growing around 120cm tall and forming extensive clumps by means of its aggressively spreading rhizomes. Considered to be a noxious weed in many areas of the tropics, it is sometimes harvested from the wild for its wide range of edible, medicinal and other uses. It is sometimes used in soil stabilization schemes.

Local uses: The flowers and the roots are antibacterial, diuretic, febrifuge, sialagogue, styptic and tonic. The flowers are used in the treatment of haemorrhages, wounds etc. They are decocted and used to treat urinary tract infections, fevers, thirst etc. A Barefoot Doctors Manual.

Chemical constituent: The plant contains the triterpenoids arundoin, cylindrin and fernenol (Var. koenigii, Nishimoto, Ito and Natori, 1968).

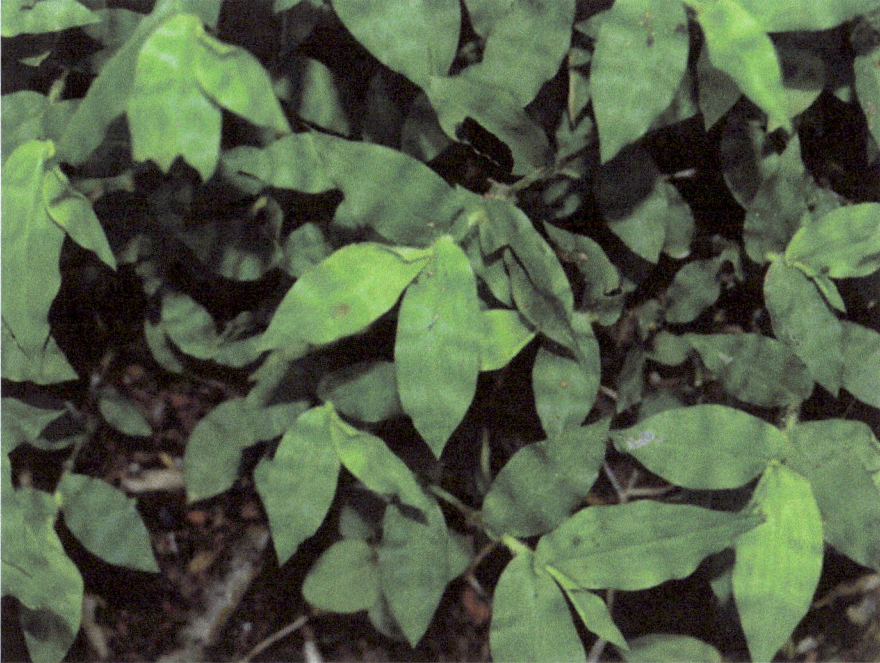

Family: Poaceae

Botanical name: *Oplismenus burmanii*

Common name: Basketgrss, wavyleaf basketgrass

History: Itcanbefoundin Floridaandon Hawaiibutisnativeto Zimbabwe. *"Oplismenus burmannii* (Retz.) P. Beauv. Burmann's basketgrass". USDA. PLANTS Profile

Local uses: Variegated forms have been cultivated as house plants in Europe. Locally occurring species in Australia have been used for revegetation and reclamation in shady or wet areas, though some can be invasive. Some have been promoted as local native plants for wildlife gardens, and as lawn grass. They are edible to livestock. Scholz, Ursula (1981). Monograph of the genus Oplismenus.

Chemical constituent: Hytosterol glucosides; Acylated phytosterol glucosides; 3a-Clionasterol glucoside; Acylated 3b-clionasterol glucosides.

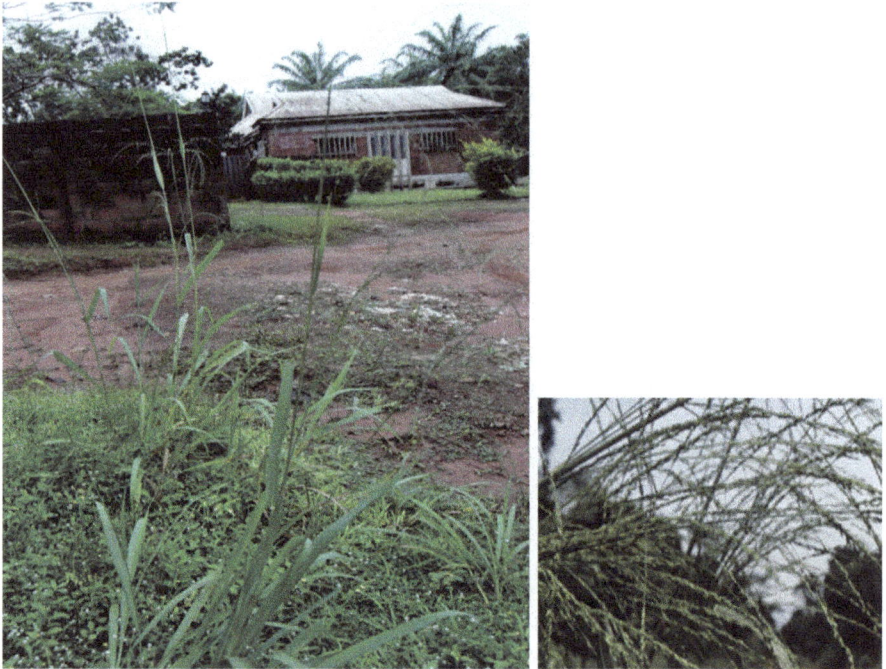

Family: Poaceae

Botanical name: *Panicum maximum*

Common name: Guinea grass

History: Guinea grass is East African in origin, but is now widely culti-vated throughout the tropics and subtropics as a forage. It was introduced from Africa into the West Indies before 1756, but for production of bird seed rather than forage. It reached Singapore in 1876 and the Philippines in 1907 and is now widely distributed throughout South-East Asia.

Local uses: Guinea grass is a palatable and good quality tropical grass used as forage for ruminants in grazed pastures or in cut-and-carry systems. Guinea grass forage is also dried and ground for use in mixtures with le-gumes as leaf meal, mainly for non-ruminants such as chickens and pigs. It can be conserved as hay or ensiled. It is also used as medicine for heartburn by the Malays under the name "berita" Van Oudtshoorn, F. 1999. Guide to grasses of southern Africa. Briza Publications, Pretoria.

Chemical constituents: The forage is reported to contain 5.9 g pro-tein, 1.6 g fat, 81.9 g total carbohydrate, 35.7 g fiber, 10.6 g ash, 2090 mg Ca, and 590 mg P (Duke and Atchley, 1984).

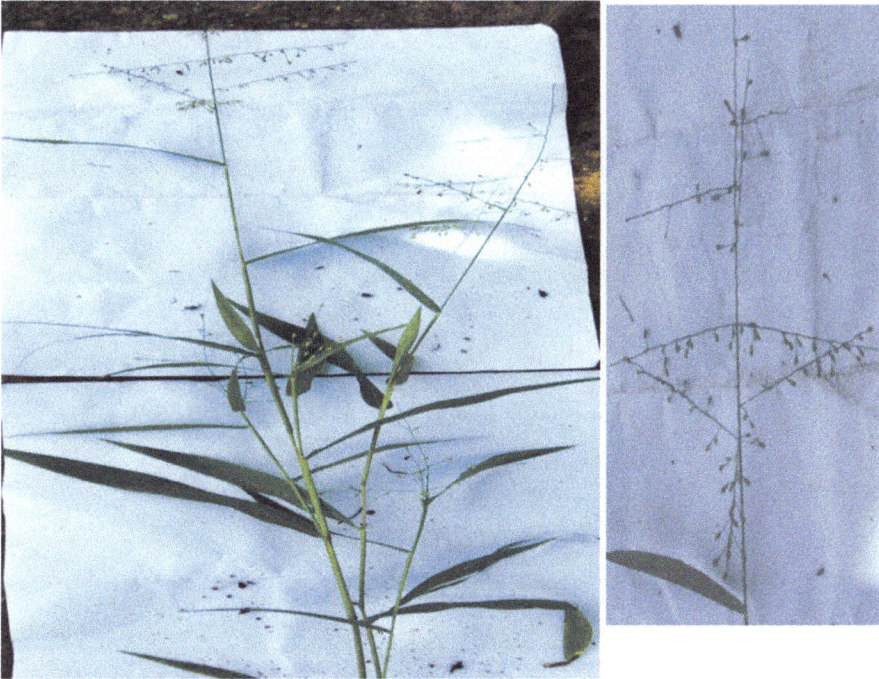

Family: Poaceae

Botanical name: *Panicum latifolium*

Common name: Panicgrass

History: Panicum (panicgrass) is a large genus of about 450 species of grasses native throughout the tropical regions of the world, with a few species extending into the northern temperate zone. They are often large, annual or perennial grasses, growing to 1–3 m tall. "Panicum". Natural Resources Conservation Service PLANTS Database.

Local uses: The smoke of the burning plant is used to fumigate wounds and as a disinfectant in the treatment of smallpox and throat infections. Glossary of Indian Medicinal Plants

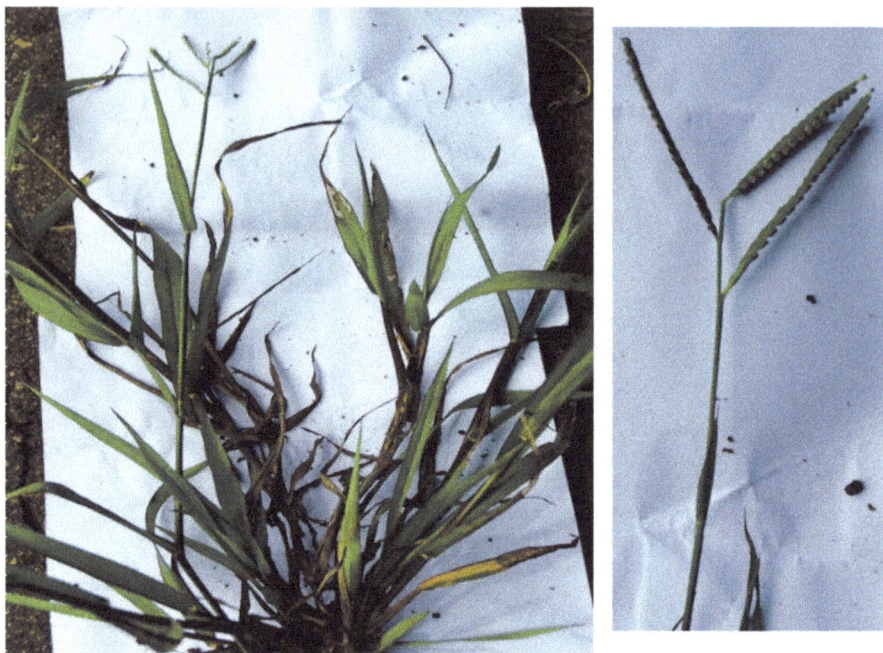

Family: *Poaceae*

Botanical name: *Paspalum scrobiculatum*

Common name: The kodo millet, cow grass, rice grass, ditch millet.

History: *Paspalum scrobiculatum,* Kodo millet is an annual grain that is grown in primarily in India, but also in the Philippines, Indonesia, Vietnam, Thailand, and in West Africa where it originates. It is grown as a minor crop in most of these areas, with the exception of the Deccan plateau in India where it is grown as a major food source. It is a very hardy crop that is drought tolerant and can survive on marginal soils where other crops may not survive and can supply 450–900 kg of grain per hectare. Kodo millet has large potential to provide nourishing food to subsistence farmers in Africa and elsewhere.

Local uses: Widely cultivated as a minor millet in Africa and Asia, especially India (Senthivel et al., 1994; Anon., 1996; Ramasamy *et al.,* 1996). Also used for forage (Bisset *et al.,* 1974; Kitamura and Nada, 1986; Su and Lin, 1994; Compere et al., 1995) and as a feed supplement (Kapoor *et al.,* 1987). In India, it has been used as a substrate for mushroom production (Kumar and Chandra, 1998) and for medicinal purposes (Roy and Pal, 1994).

Chemical constituents: The grain is composed of 11% of protein, providing 9 grams/100 g consumed. It is an excellent source of fibre at 10 grams (37-38%), as opposed to rice, which provides 0.2/100 g, and wheat, which provides 1.2/100 g. An adequate fibre source helps combat the feeling of hunger. Kodo millet contains 66.6 g of carbohydrates and 353 kcal per 100 g of grain, comparable to other millets. It also contains 3.6 g of fat per 100 g. It provides minimal amounts of iron, at 0.5/100 mg, and minimal amounts of calcium, and 27/100 mg. Kodo millets also contain high amounts of polyphenols, an antioxidant compound. "Millets: Future of Food & Farming". Millet Network of India.

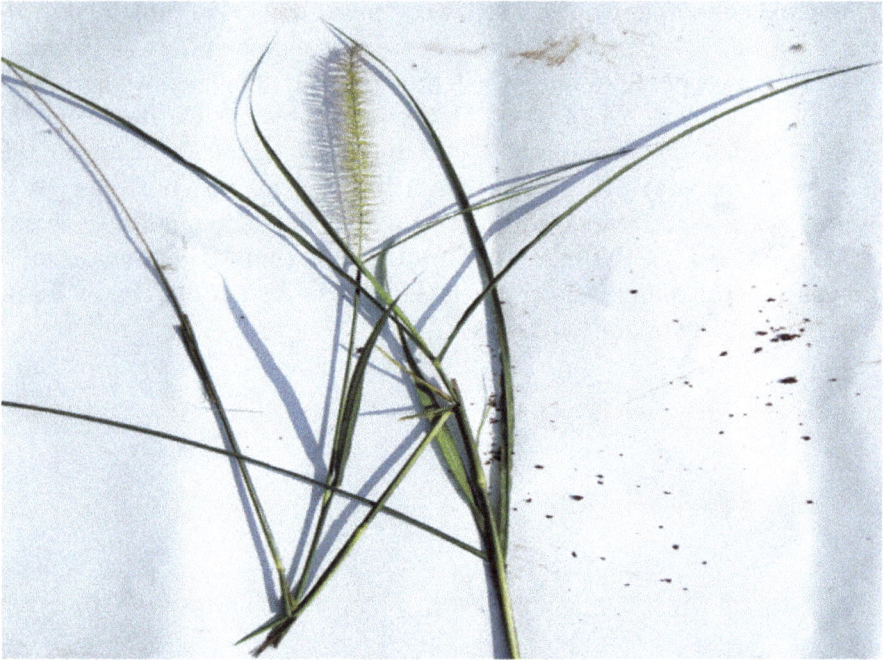

Family: Poaceae

Botanical name: *Pennisetum purpureum*

Common name: Napier grass, elephant grass or Uganda grass

History: A species of perennial tropical grass native to the African grasslands. Historically, this wild species has been used primarily for grazing

Local uses: It is more affordable for farmers than insecticide use. In addition to this, Napier grasses improve soil fertility, and protect arid land from soil erosion. It is also utilized for firebreaks, windbreaks, in paper pulp production and most recently to produce bio-oil, biogas and charcoal.

Chemical constituents: Trace of alkaloid in the leaves.

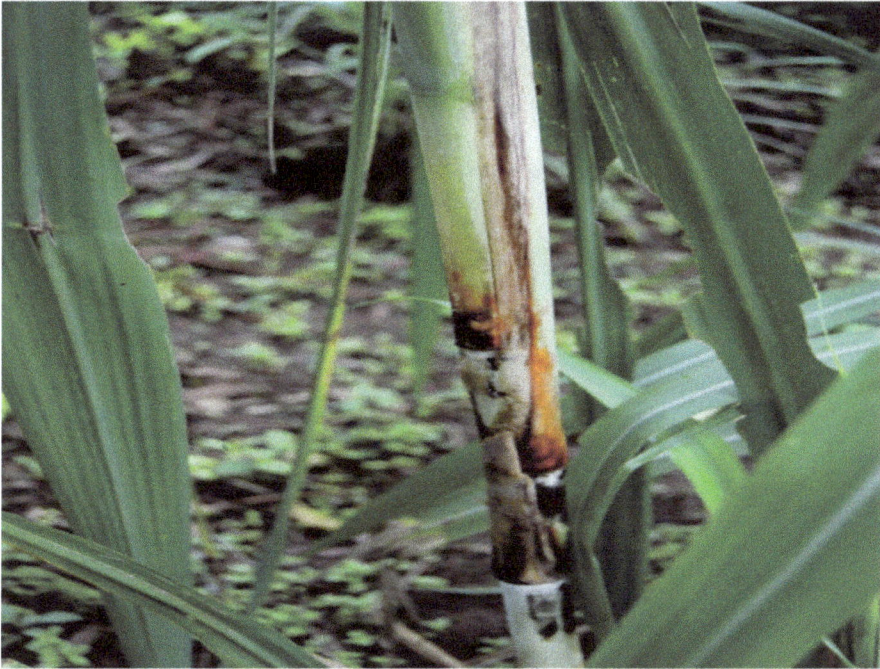

Family: Poaceae

Botanical name: *Saccharium officinalis*

Common name: Sugarcane

Local name: Benin: Ukhure, ***Hausa:*** Reke

History: It originated in southeast Asia and is now cultivated in tropical and subtropical countries worldwide for the production of sugar and other products.

Local uses: Portions of the stem of this and several other species of sugarcane have been used from ancient times for chewing to extract the sweet juice. *S. officinarum* and its hybrids are grown for the production of sugar, ethanol, and other industrial uses in tropical and subtropical regions around the world. The stems and the by products of the sugar industry are used for feeding to livestock. As its specific name (officinarum, "of dispensaries") implies, it is also used in traditional medicine both internally and externally.

Chemical constituents: Contains sucrose (glucose and fructose) in juice, cellulose (many glucose units) in the fibre.

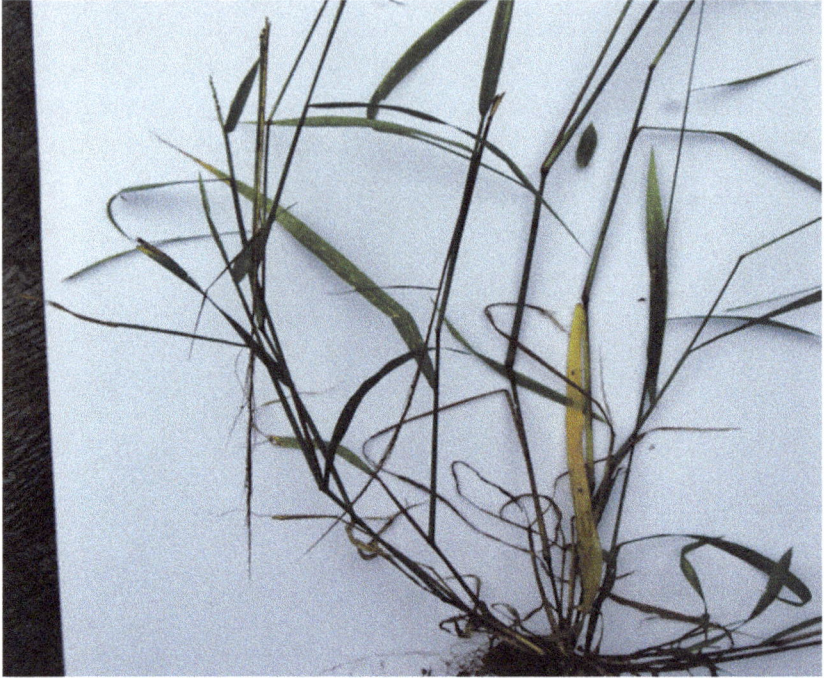

Family: Poaceae

Botanical name: *Seteria longiseta*

History: Three species of Setaria have been domesticated and used as staple crops throughout foxtail millet *(S. italica),* korali *(S. pumila)* in India, and, before the full domestication of maize, *Setaria macrostachya* in Mexico. Several species are still cultivated today as food or as animal fodder, such as foxtail millet *(S. italica)* and korali *(S. pumila),* while others are considered invasive weeds. *Setaria viridis* is currently being developed as a genetic model system for bioenergy grasses.

Local uses: In Kenya, increasingly grown as forage grass in recent time.

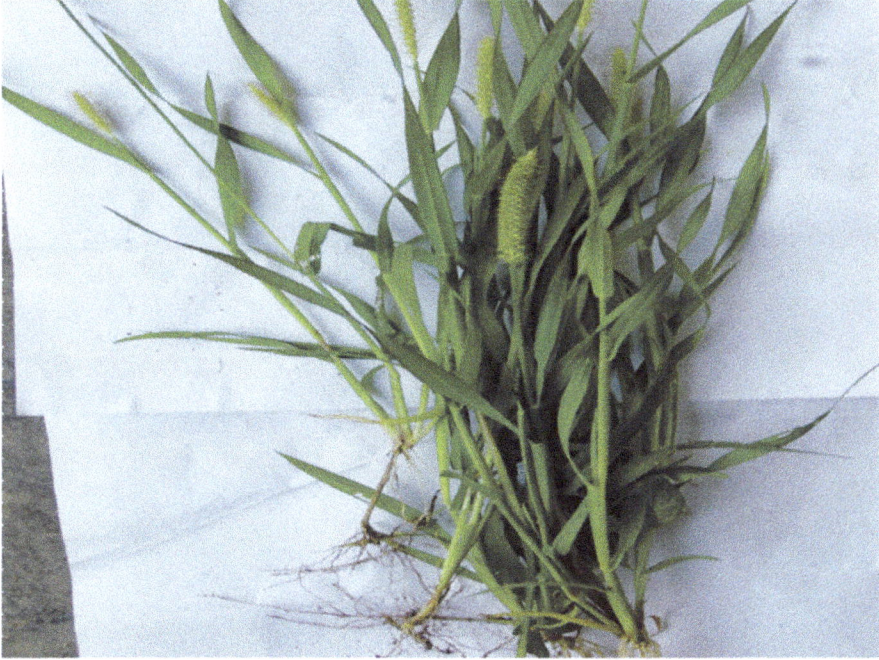

Family: Poaceae

Botanical name: *Seteria pumila*

History: It is native to Europe and Africa but it is known throughout the world as a common weed. It grows in lawns, sidewalks, roadsides, cultivated fields, and many other places.

Local uses: The grass can be made into a good hay. In Lesotho, sheaves of grain are tied together using rope made from culms of *S. pumila* that are twisted together. In some areas this grass plays an important role in stabilising bare soil to protect it from erosion. It can also be eaten as a sweet or savoury food in all the ways that rice is used, or ground into a powder and made into porridge, cakes, puddings.

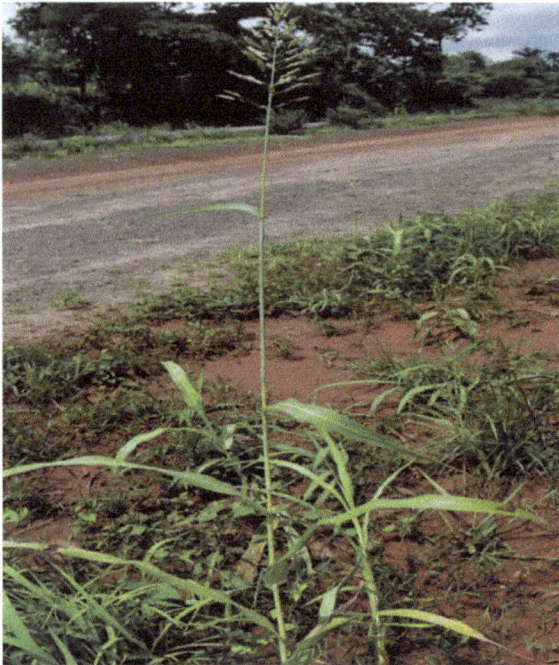

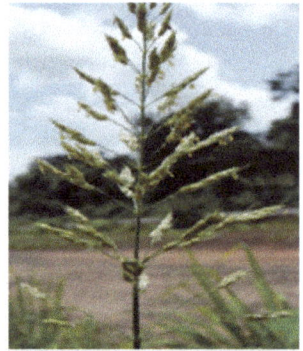

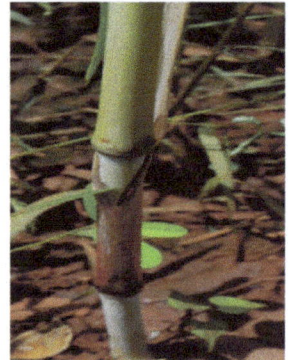

Family: Poaceae

Botanical name: *Sorghum bicolor*

History: Sorghum originated in northern Africa and is now cultivated widely in tropical and subtropical regions.

Local uses: Sorghum is the world's fifth most important cereal crop after rice, wheat, maize and barley. It is also used for making a traditional corn broom. Sorghum is one of a number of grains used as wheat substitutes in gluten-free recipes and products. It is used in feed and pasturage for live-stock.

Chemical constituents: Hydroxybenzoic acids gallic acid flavones Apigenin, flavanones, naringen flavonols

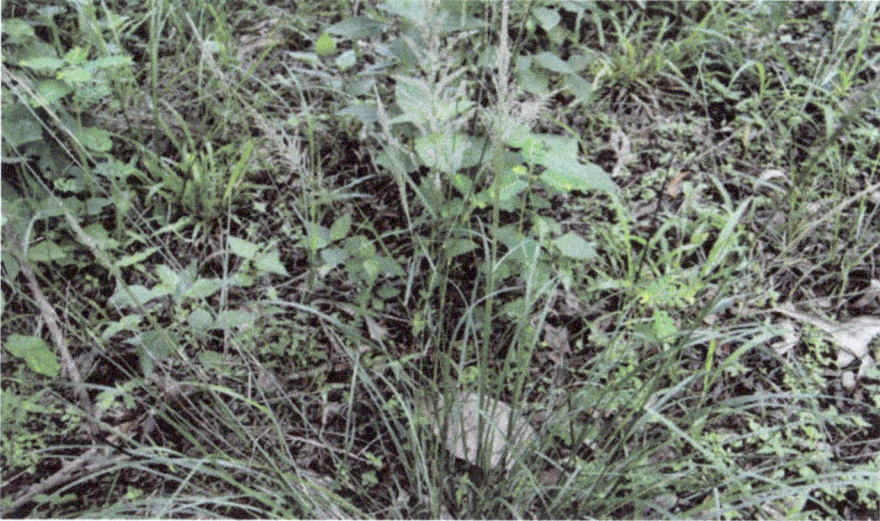

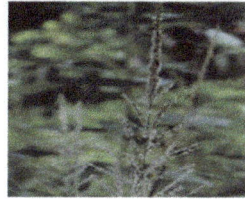

Family: Poaceae

Botanical name: *Sporobolus indicus*

History: This bunch grass is native to temperate and tropical areas of the Americas. It can be found in more regions, as well as on many Pacific Islands, as an introduced species and a common weed of disturbed habitat.

Local uses: It is considered to be an antifertility drug in some countries. A fibre is obtained from the leaves. The tough culms are used for making hats and other items that can be woven from straw.

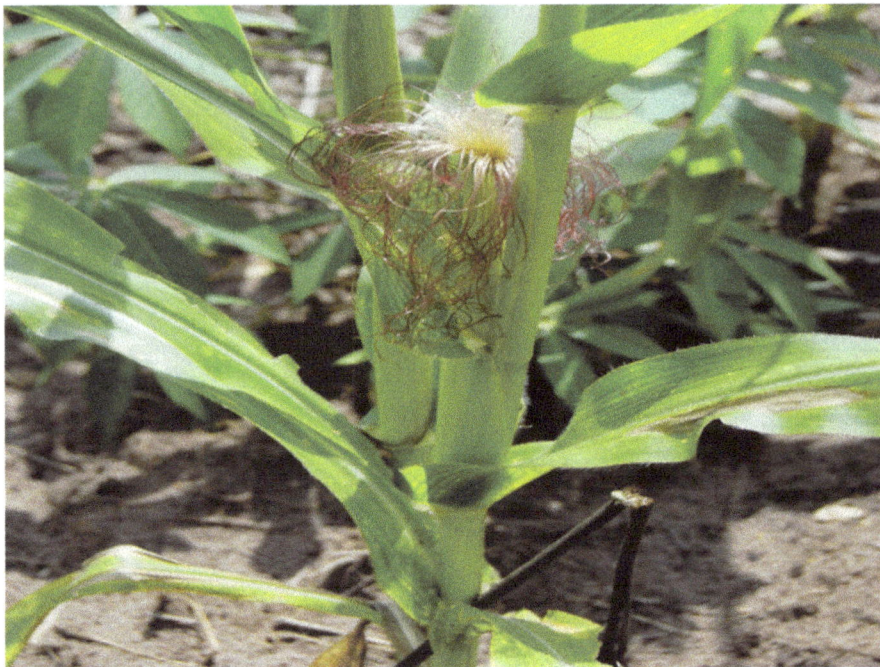

Family: Poaceae **Botanical name:** *Zee mays*

Common name: Maize

Local name: *Yoruba:* Agbado, *Igbo:* Oka *Hausa:* Masara

History: Maize is an erect, robust, usually unbranched annual plant. It can grow up to 6 metres tall but is usually around 2 metres with cultivars that can range from around 1 metre up to 3 metres or more. A common crop around the world, providing a range of foods including popcorn, sweetcorn and can be ground into a flour. First domesticated in the Americas around 4,000 BC.

Local uses: The mature seed can be dried and used whole or ground into a flour. It has a very mild flavour and is used especially as a thickening agent in foods such as custards. The dried seed of certain varieties can be heated in an oven when they burst to make Popcorn. The seed can also be sprouted and used in making uncooked breads and cereals. The fresh succulent 'silks' (the flowering parts of the cob) can also be eaten. The pollen is used as an ingredient of soups. The seed is diuretic and a mild stimulant. It is a good emollient poultice for ulcers, swellings and rheumatic pains, and is widely used in the treatment of cancer, tumours and warts. Medicinal Plants of China. Duke. J. A. and Ayensu. E. S. (1985)

Chemical constituents: *The protein that is rich in* proline, glutamine, leucine and/or alanine.

References

A Barefoot Doctors Manual. Running Press ISBN 0-914294-92-X Bisset *et al.*, 1974; Kitamura and Nada, 1986; Su and Lin, 1994; Compere et al., 1995

DeFilipps, R. A.; Maina, S. L.; & Crepin, J. Duke and Atchley, (1984)

Duke. J. A. and Ayensu. E. S. Medicinal Plants of China Reference Publications, Inc. ISBN 0-917256-20-4 (1985-00-00)

Duke. J. (1983)

Galinato M., Moody K., Piggin C. M. (1999)

Glossary of Indian Medicinal Plants (Including the Supplement). Chopra. R. N., Nayar. S. L. and Chopra. I. C.

Handbook of Energy Crops. Duke. J. (1983)

Handbook of Energy Crops. Duke. J. (1983)

Heuzé V., Tran G., Giger-Reverdin S., 2015. Scrobic (Paspalum scrobiculatum) forage and grain. Feedipedia, a programme by INRA, CIRAD, AFZ and FAO. https://www.feedipedia.org/ node/401http://botany.si.edu/bdg/medicinal/index.html http:// ecocrop.fao.org/ecocrop/srv/en/home http://ecocrop.fao.org/ ecocrop/srv/en/home http://onlinelibrary.wiley.com/doi/10.1002/ jccs.201300484/epdf?r3_referer=wol&tracking_action=preview_ click&show_ checkout=1&purchase_referrer=www.google.com. ng&purchase_ site_license=LICENSE_DENIED http://www. fao.org/ag/AGP/AGPC/doc/Gbase/Default.htm http://www. iucnredlist.org/

Kapoor et al., 1987 McDonald, (1981)

Medicinal Plants of China. Duke. J. A. and Ayensu. E. S. (1985) Millets. Earth360. (2010-13). http://earth360.in/web/Millets. html

Millets: Future of Food & Farming". Millet Network of India. (No date given, accessed November 13th 2013.) http://www.swaraj. org/ shikshantar/millets.pdf

Orskov, E.R. 1982 Protein Nutrition in Ruminants. Academic Press, London. Pages 735–752, doi:10.1016/0040-4020(68)88023-8\ Panicum. Natural Resources Conservation Service PLANTS Database.USDA. Retrieved 15 May 2015.

Prawirodigdo (1985)

Rothauge, (2014) Roy and Pal, 1994

Ruffo, C.K.: Birnie, A. & Tengnas, B. (2002)

Samarakoon et al., 1990

Scholz, Ursula (1981). Monograph of the genus Oplismenus.

Senthivel et al., 1994; Anon., 1996; Ramasamy et al., 1996

The Useful Plants of West Tropical Africa. Burkil. H. M. (1985 – 2004) The Useful Plants of West Tropical Africa. Burkil. H. M. (1985 – 2004) The Useful Plants of West Tropical Africa. Burkil. H. M. (1985 – 2004) The Useful Plants of West Tropical Africa. Burkil. H. M. (1985 – 2004) The New RHS Dictionary of Gardening. Huxley. A. (1992.)

US Forest Service, 2011; FAO, 2011; Quattrocchi, 2006; Cook et al., 2005 USDA. PLANTS Profile. Retrieved May 14, 2013

Van Oudtshoorn, F. 1999. Guide to grasses of southern Africa. Briza Publications, Pretoria.

Veldkamp J.F (1996)

Index

12, 13, 17, 21, 22, 30, 31, 52,
56, 57, 76, 85, 97, 153
Tridax 129

V

Velvet 53

W

Whiteberry 93
Wild cocoyam 114
Wild gourd 118
Windmill grass 140

Y

Yellow cassia 61
Yellow mombin 62
Yellow yam 124

www.ingramcontent.com/pod-product-compliance
Lightning Source LLC
Chambersburg PA
CBHW040141270326
41928CB00022B/3282